The Aging Mouth

Frontiers of Oral Physiology

Vol. 6

Series Editor
D. B. Ferguson, Manchester

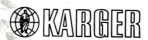

Basel · München · Paris · London · New York · New Delhi · Singapore · Tokyo · Sydney

The Aging Mouth

Volume Editor
D. B. Ferguson, Manchester

61 figures and 15 tables, 1987

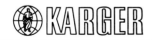

Basel · München · Paris · London · New York · New Delhi · Singapore · Tokyo · Sydney

Frontiers of Oral Physiology

Library of Congress Cataloging-in-Publication Data
The Aging mouth.
(Frontiers of oral physiology; vol. 6)
Includes bibliographies and index.
1. Mouth – Aging. I. Ferguson, D.B. II. Series.
[DNLM: 1. Aging – physiology. 2. Dental Pulp – physiology.
3. Jaw – physiology. 4. Mouth – physiology. 5. Taste – physiology.
W1 FR946GP v. 6 / WI 200 A267]
QP146.A35 1987 612′.31 87-3316
ISBN 3–8055–4513–4

Drug Dosage
The authors and the publisher have exerted every effort to ensure that drug selection and dosage set forth in this text are in accord with current recommendations and practice at the time of publication. However, in view of ongoing research, changes in government regulations, and the constant flow of information relating to drug therapy and drug reactions, the reader is urged to check the package insert for each drug for any change in indications and dosage and for added warnings and precautions. This is particularly important when the recommended agent is a new and/or infrequently employed drug.

© Copyright 1987 by S. Karger AG, P.O. Box, CH-4009 Basel (Switzerland)
Printed in Switzerland by Thür AG Offsetdruck, Pratteln
ISBN 3-8055-4513-4

Contents

Oral Metabolic Changes in Older Subjects

Changes in Salivary Function in Older Subjects

Changes in Oral Sensory Function in Older Subjects

Aging and Chemosensory Perception

Taste Perception Mechanisms

Front. oral Physiol., vol. 6, pp. 1–6 (Karger, Basel 1987)

An Overview of Physiological Changes in the Aging Mouth

D. B. Ferguson

University of Manchester, Department of Physiology, Manchester, England

Introduction

With increasing interest among the research community in the effects and problems of aging, and an awareness among medical and dental practitioners that older age groups constitute a growing proportion of the population, there has developed a need for readily accessible sources of information on the biology of aging in the human. In the medical field such sources are available: in dentistry there are now two journals devoted to gerodontology. This chapter and the book as a whole aim to present an overview of the normal process of aging in key oral tissues. They provide a basis for, but do not extend onwards to, considerations of pathological changes in the mouths of older subjects, whether these be due to disease, neoplasia, or medical or dental treatment.

Connective Tissues – Bone, Dental Pulp and Dental Hard Tissues

The connective tissues of the mouth age as do connective tissues in the rest of the body. Changes in bone with aging have been studied by many workers. Loss of calcified tissue, particularly in women, has been extensively studied and there are several reports in the literature on investigations of this in the mandible [1, 6, 11, 16, 17]. Thus, Henrikson and Wallenius [11] reported that the density of mandibular bone decreased from 1.9 to 1.5 between the ages of 45 and 90, and that throughout this age range values were 8% lower in women. Loss of calcified tissue from the mandible was directly related to that elsewhere (the radius being used as a typical control bone). In addition to being less dense the bone is often more brittle. Shapiro et al. [17] state that lamina dura is often lost and the cortical bone at the angle of mandible thinner. Atkinson and Hallsworth [1] demonstrated an increase in porosity of bone with aging. This was mainly due to an increase in vascular spaces. Although the volume occupied by each canaliculus stayed constant or even increased, the total canalicular volume decreased. Lacunar volume increased despite a reduction in the number of lacunae. Bernick et al. [6] found diffuse calcification in the bony canals, but the lacunae were filled with a glycoprotein material staining differently from that in young bone and there was a decrease in the number of osteocytes and osteones. The walls of the blood capillaries supplying the bone thickened with age. In addition to changes in the distribution of calcium salts, the blood supply to older bone may be impaired and the active cells of bone reduced in number. Changes also occur in the collagen matrix leading to greater cross-linkage and the replacement of reducible cross-links by non-reducible and acid-stable cross-links. These are discussed in the next section of this book by Shikata et al. In addition to the previously reported pyridinoline cross-links they describe a new cross-link, histidinoalanine, and suggest that both these molecules increase in concentration in mandibular bone as it ages.

The dental pulp is another connective tissue. It, too, shows signs of aging. These include a reduction in size and volume, a decrease in cell numbers, an increase in number and thickness of collagen fibres, the presence of calcified masses and a decrease in the number of blood and lymphatic vessels. These are described in this volume by Bernick and then a more detailed account of the collagen changes is given by Neilson. The amount of collagen in the pulp actually decreases with age although the aggregation of fine fibrils into larger fibrils and the diminution in pulp size give an impression that the amount is increasing. The rate of synthesis decreases and there is more cross-link formation. The amount of dihydroxyl lysinonorleucine in dental pulps increases with age. The dental pulp collagen is mainly types I and III: in animals the proportion of type III increases with age. Fried [this volume] looks at another aspect of aging in the pulp: the changes in its innervation. These affect not only the pulp, but also the dentine, since it is from the pulp that dentine receives its innervation. After summarizing the changes seen in the dental tissues generally Fried describes the gradual loss of nerve fibres from the tooth as it ages and the development and thickening of perineural sheaths about the nerves.

The changes in the dental hard tissues which occur as the teeth age have been recognised for many years and most textbooks of dental anatomy describe these in some detail. The aging of dental enamel, dentine and cementum will not therefore be described here.

Salivary Glands and Saliva

However, the changes in the salivary glands and the saliva they produce have only recently been investigated. Morphologically, changes in salivary glands have been known for many years. Drummond [this volume] describes these generally and then gives an account specifically of minor labial and lingual glands. Scott then reviews his own observations on submandibular and sublingual glands. In summary, the aging glands appear less compact, with the acini occupying a smaller proportion of the gland volume, the ducts occupying an increased proportion, and fibrous and fibro-adipose tissue making up a larger proportion. Cells with many mitochondria, found in association with the ducts, and termed oncocytes, increase in number as salivary glands grow older and there is an increase in the incidence of focal obstructive adenitis. Biochemical studies of salivary glands show that, as in other tissues, rates of protein biosynthesis decrease with age. There are changes in the molecules present but the reasons for these changes are unclear. Kim [this volume] points out that the rate of production of secretory proteins may be reduced by the slowing down of secretory activity in the glands. However, there are reports of changes in the types of protein secreted: acid DNAse activity is reduced, sialic acid content decreases, and some isoenzymes of α-amylase exhibit greater electrophoretic mobility but reduced enzyme activity. In the final paper of this section, Baum emphasises that most studies of salivary function in older individuals have concentrated on flow rate and have been inadequately controlled as to the state of health and medication of the subjects. In normal, healthy, non-medicated subjects salivary secretion does not change with age. The composition does change: the observations of Baum et al. [5] show that sodium concentration is lower, whilst those of Chauncey et al. [7] show decreases in chloride and total protein concentrations also.

Oral Sensory Function – Taste

Oral sensory mechanisms and oral motor control may also be affected by aging. Older subjects not uncommonly complain that foods do not taste as they used to. This may be due to changes in the foods or the diet themselves, but equally may be due to changes in taste sensation either at the receptors or in the central nervous system. It has been known for many years that the number of taste buds declines with age [2]. Although more recent work [3] questions this, such a decline could affect sensitivity to all taste sensations or result in selective loss of sensation. Weiffenback [this volume] discusses this question and comments particularly on the methods of measuring taste performance and the significance of the results. He points out that the effects of aging on detection of different taste stimuli vary and that perception of increments of taste stimuli may also be affected. Murphy extends the discussion by concentrating on the perception of taste stimuli. This involves the interaction of taste and olfactory stimuli (and also texture appreciation) and the association of emotional reactions – whether taste stimuli are perceived as pleasant or unpleasant. Data are presented which demonstrate differences in perception of so-called basic tastes when presented in water or in beverages or foodstuffs. Nutritional state also appears to influence taste appreciation.

Weiffenbach et al. [19] show that thresholds for sweet and acid are not affected by aging, but those for salt and bitter are. The response to increasing concentrations, however, declined up to at least age 40.

Oral Motor Function – Mastication, Deglutition and Speech

Three aspects of oral motor function have been studied – mastication, swallowing, and speech. Mastication has been assessed by sieving of chewed carrot either after a fixed number of masticatory strokes (the standardised 40 stroke masticatory performance test) or at the point when normal mastication produced comminution to a level deemed by the subject as appropriate for swallowing (the swallowing threshold performance test index) [8, 10, 15]. The data reported show that both these measures are affected primarily by the state of the dentition and that the performance of older subjects differs little from that of younger subjects with similar numbers of teeth or with similar dentures [9]. This contrasts with Kaplan's [14] statement that biting force reduces from 300 lb/in² to 50 lb/in² with age – although no data is given to support this. Baum and Bodner [4] found that lip seal was less efficient in older subjects. Swallowing has been examined radiographically and electromyographically. More recently ultrasound has been used. In a small group of subjects Sonies et al. [18] reported that swallowing time was increased by 25–50% in subjects over age 55. The evidence on oral motor function is therefore conflicting and more data are needed.

Speech

Although speech may be affected by changes in respiration, and in the tissues of the larynx and pharynx, as subjects age, the process of articulation in the mouth is relatively little affected [13]. In healthy subjects the main identifying feature of older speech is an increase in the fundamental frequency [12]. In this area of research, as in others, it is important that a distinction is made between subjects who are considered to be in normal health and those with possible impairment of function by disease or drugs. The criteria for classification of a subject as normal must be specified.

Conclusions

Although biochemical and morphological changes in oral tissues have been demonstrated to occur with aging, changes in normal functioning are less well documented. Most studies of healthy non-medicated subjects show little change with age. Evidence from aging subjects where health and medication have not been assessed or reported shows changes to occur but these cannot be seen as specifically age-associated. There is still a need for studies of the physiology of aging in relation to the oral cavity and its functions but these studies must be more closely controlled so as to allow evaluation of the separate influences of health, medication, the use of prosthetic appliances and aging itself. Understanding of the physiological changes is important in assessing the health of subjects and in identifying reasons for departures from the normal.

References

1 Atkinson, P. J.; Hallsworth, A. S.: The changing pore structure of aging human mandibular bone. Gerodontology 2: 57–66 (1983).

2 Avey, L. B.; Tremaine, M. J.; Monzingo, F. L.: The numerical and topographical relations of taste buds to circumvallate papillae throughout the life span. Anat. Rec. 64: 9–25 (1935).

3 Arvidson, K.: Location and variation in number of taste buds in human fungiform papillae. Scand. J. dent. Res. 87: 435–442 (1979).

4 Baum, B. J.; Bodner, L.: Aging and oral motor function; evidence for altered performance among older persons. J. dent. Res. 62: 2–6 (1983).

5 Baum, B. J.; Costa, P. T., Jr.; Izutsu, K. T.: Alteration in sodium handling by human parotid glands during aging: failure to support a simple two-stage secretion model. Am. J. Physiol. 246: R35–39 (1984).

6 Bernick, S.; Sobin, S. S.; Paule, W. J.: Changes in the microvasculature and interstitium of aged human mandibles and maxillae. Gerodontology 2: 9–14 (1983).

7 Chauncey, H. H.; Borkan, G. A.; Wayler, A. M.; Feller, R. P.; Kapur, K. K.: Parotid fluid composition in healthy aging males. Adv. Physiol. Sci. 28: 323–328 (1981).

8 Chauncey, H. H.; Kapur, K. K.; Feller, R. P.; Wayler, A. H.: Altered masticatory function and perceptual estimates of chewing experience Spe, Care Dent. 1: 250–256 (1981).

9 Feldman, R. S.; Alman, J.; Muench, M. E.; Chauncey, H. H.: Longitudinal stability and masticatory function of human dentition. Gerodontology 3: 107–113 (1984).

10 Feldman, R. S.; Kapur, K.; Alman, J. E.; Chauncey, H. H.: Aging and mastication: changes in performance and in the swallowing threshold with natural dentition. J. Am. Geriat. Soc. 28: 97–103 (1980).

11 Henrikson, P. A.; Wallenius, K.: The mandible and osteoporosis. J. oral Rehabil. 1: 67–84 (1974).

12 Harii, Y.; Ryan. W. J.: Fundamental frequency characteristics and perceived age of adult male speakers. Folia phoniat. 33: 227–231 (1981).

13 Kahane, J. C.: Anatomic and physiologic changes in aging peripheral speech mechanism; in Beasley, Davis, Aging: communication processes and disorders, chap. 2, pp. 21–45 (Grune & Stratton, New York 1981).

14 Kaplan, H.: The oral cavity in geriatrics. Geriatrics 26: 96–102 (1971).

15 Kapur, K. K.; Somon, S.: Masticatory performance and efficiency in denture wearers. J. prosth. Dent. 14: 687–694 (1964).

16 Kribbs, P. J.; Chesnut, C. H.; Smith, D. E.: Oral findings in osteoporosis. J. prosth. dent. 50: 576–579, 719–724 (1983).

17 Shapiro, S.; Bomberg, T. J.; Benson, B. W.; Harnby, C. I.: Post-menopausal osteoporosis: dental patients at risk. Gerodontics 1: 220–225 (1985).

18 Sonies, B. C.; Stone, M.; Shawker, T.: Speech and swallowing in the elderly. Gerodontology 2: 115–123 (1984).

19 Weiffenbach, J. M.; Baum, B. J.; Burghauser, R.: Taste thresholds: quality specific variations with human aging. J. Geront. 32: 372–377 (1982).

Dr. D. B. Ferguson, University of Manchester, Department of Physiology, Stopford Building, Machester M13 9PT (England)

Front. oral Physiol., vol. 6, pp. 7–30 (Karger, Basel 1987)

Age Changes to the Dental Pulp

Sol Bernick

Department of Anatomy and Cell Biology, University of Southern California,
School of Medicine, Los Angeles, Calif., USA

Introduction

The dental pulp is a loose connective tissue mass containing cells, predominantly fibroblasts, undifferentiated mesenchymal cells, macrophages, and odontoblasts. Collagen fibers and extracellular glycosaminoglycans (GAG) occupy the extracellular spaces. Blood and lymphatic vessels as well as nerves course through this connective tissue structure. During the aging process these pulpal components undergo changes similar to other structures in the oral cavity and throughout the body. However, there are specific age alterations only found in the dental pulp. Age changes which have been reported in the literature include: (1) reduction in size and volume of the pulp; (2) decrease in cellular components; (3) increase in the number and thickness of collagen fibers; (4) the presence of dystrophic calcified masses, and (5) decrease in the number of blood and lymphatic vessels and associated nerves [26]. Each of these will be discussed in this presentation.

Reduction in Size and Volume of Pulp

The pulps of non-erupted permanent teeth consist of loose connective tissue stroma which includes an odontoblastic zone adjacent to the predentine and a cell-free zone, the zone of Weil, lying between the odontoblastic layer and the pulp proper. At this stage of development, there are a few vessels and nerves in the pulp proper and zone of Weil. No nerves are demonstrable in the odontoblastic zone (fig. 1a). The pulpal tissue of erupted non-carious teeth from individuals varying in age from 20 to 45 years still consists of loose connective tissue in which the collagen fibers are small and thin. At the same time there is a rich network of vessels and nerves that traverse the root and coronal pulp (fig. 1b). In teeth obtained from individuals of both sexes over 45 years of age,

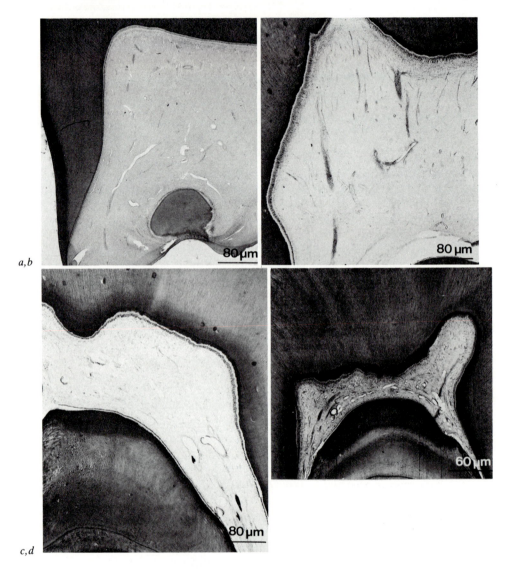

a,b

c,d

Fig. 1. a Sections of a non-erupted lower third molar obtained from a 16-year-old female. Note the beginning of root formation. The pulp chamber is wide and consists of a loose mesenchymal-like connective tissue. There is a sparsity of both blood vessels and nerves. ×20. *b* Sections of an upper molar from a young adult. Note the wide pulp chamber; the connective tissue stroma of loose connective tissue elements, and the presence of an abundant number of vessels and nerves throughout the pulp. ×20. *c* Section of an upper molar

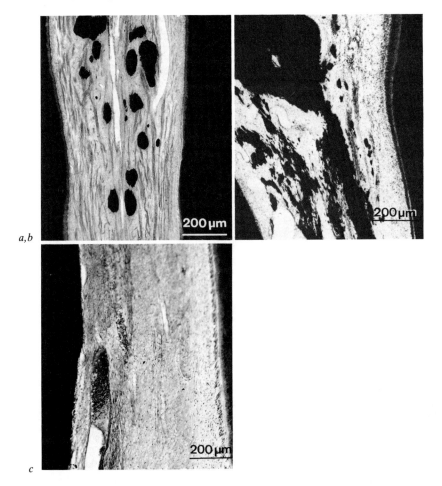

a,b

c

Fig. 2. a The root pulp from a 58-year-old individual. Note the small calcified bodies scattered throughout the root pulp. ×50. *b* The root pulp of an upper first molar from an individual more than 50 years of age. Notice the heavy diffuse calcification throughout the root. ×50. *c* The root pulp from a molar tooth of a 15-year-old male. Note that the pulpal connective tissue is free of dystrophic calcification. ×50. All sections were stained with iron hematoxylin.

from a 60-year-old male. In comparison to the preceding illustrations, there is a narrowing of the pulp chamber as a result of continual deposition of dentine both occlusally and in the furcation regions. ×20. *d* Section of an upper molar from an individual over 65 years of age. Note that the narrowness of the pulp chamber is the result of a progressive apposition of dentin in the furcation area. ×15. All sections were stained with PAS-hematoxylin.

there is a progressive reduction in pulpal area (fig 1c, d). The basic reduction in the coronal pulpal area is the result of a continual apposition of
dentine occlusally as well as at the furcation region. Although most text
books in oral histology describe only the occlusal dentine deposition as
the causative factor in the diminution of pulpal size, it is apparent that the
deposition of dentine at the furcation area is greater than that of occusal
dentine (fig. 1d).

Presences of Dystrophic Calcification

The presence of dystrophic calcified bodies in the pulps of teeth is a
common feature of old teeth from individuals over the age of 45 years.
They are located in the root pulp, coronal pulp, or both. In a previous
study by the author [3] 90% of the 'old' pulps exhibited diffuse calcified
bodies. This percentage is similar to that found by Hill [17]. These calcified bodies or masses are not true dentinal pulpstones. They are usually
first seen in the root pulp as isolated small calcified bodies (fig. 2a). In
other teeth multiple larger masses are observed that may apparently
obliterate the root canal (fig. 2b). On the other hand, there are no indications of dystrophic calcified bodies or masses in 'young' teeth (fig. 2c).
Figure 3a illustrates the extension of the calcifying process from the root
to the coronal pulp. The isolated masses coalesce to form larger masses
that fuse with the dentine (fig. 3b). The calcified masses in the coronal
pulp may become larger in size and fuse together to obliterate the normal
pulp architecture (fig. 3c). In addition it should be mentioned that there is
a direct association of these masses with collagen fibers (fig. 3d). Milch
[22] postulated that with increased cross-linkage of collagen during
advancing age there is an enhanced tendency for these fibers to become
mineralized. It was noted in our study [5] that the collagen bundles of the
vascular and neural sheaths of the younger pulps stained blue with Alcian
blue-PAS combination whereas in the old pulp they were Schiff-positive.
The Schiff-positive fibers were the nuclei for mineralization. None of the
young teeth examined exhibited any sites of mineralization in either the
root or the coronal pulp.

Decrease in Number of Cells

The cellular composition of the human pulp is modified during the
aging process. Frolich [12] has shown that the number of cells are reduced
by 50% in aged pulps. In aging rats, for example, there was a loss of 75%

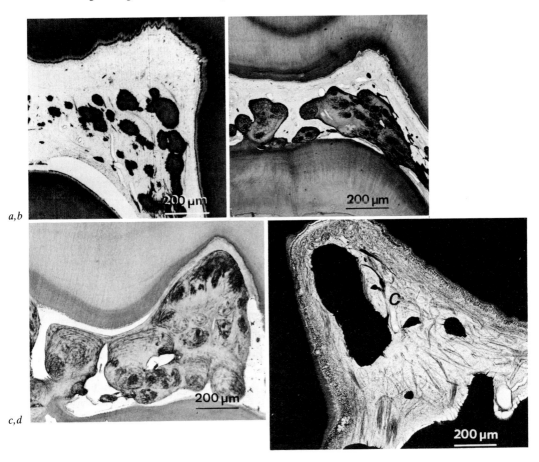

Fig. 3. *a* Section of an 'old' molar tooth. Note the process of dystrophic calcification has extended from the root pulp into the coronal chamber. ×50. *b* Coronal pulp chamber of an 'old' tooth. The isolated calcified bodies have coalesced into larger masses. Note that the masses have joined together and have fused onto the dentine. ×50. *c* Section of an 'old' tooth. The calcified bodies have fused to form a large mass that has ankylosed with the dentine at the cuspal area. ×50. *d* A section of the pulp from an 'old' tooth. Note that the collagen fibers (C) form the loci for dystrophic calcification. ×50. All sections were stained with iron hematoxyl in.

of the cells in comparison with 'young' pulps [24]. The kinetics of rat molar pulp cells at various ages was investigated by Pinzon et al. [23]. They reported that there was a significant decrease in the number of regenerating cells with increasing age.

Fibroblasts show degeneration with increasing age as characterized by small size and a decrease in the number of organelles including the rough endoplasmic reticulum, mitochondria, and Golgi complex [16]. Odontoblasts also exhibit degeneration with age. Ultrastructural studies reveal an increase in vacuole numbers and gradual degenerative changes leading to the absence of cells over some or all of the pulpal surfaces [8]. From about the age of 20 years, cells gradually decrease in number until the age of 70 when the cell density has decreased by about half [29]. Figure 4a illustrates the odontoblastic layer from a molar tooth of a 25-year-old individual. The zone consists of multiple layers of odontoblasts. In contrast there is a marked loss of odontoblasts in the older teeth as seen in figure 4b. In this molar tooth the odontoblastic layer appears to be limited to one to three layers, and the cells are small and darkly stained. The decrease in the number of odontoblasts is parallelled by a loss of cells, including fibroblasts, in the pulp proper of 'old' teeth as observed in figure 4d. The pulps of 'young' teeth exhibited a great number of cells of contrast to the number seen in the old pulps (fig. 4c). Another result of the loss of odontoblasts was seen in the dentinal tubules. In the old teeth there is an increase in peritubular dentine, leading to a complete sclerosing of the tubule. In young teeth the tubule is lined with Alcian blue-positive material surrounding the cell extensions of the odontoblastic cell body. On the other hand, in the 'old' teeth, the walls of the dentinal tubules appear intensely red following the Alcian blue-PAS staining. Many of these tubules are completely filled with the Schiff-positive material. The obliteration of the dentinal tubules in the aged teeth is similar to what occurred in the lacunae and canaliculi of the compact bone in aged, human mandibles and maxillae [7].

Changes in Collagenous Elements

It has been reported that there is an increase in collagen elements of the pulp during the aging process [8, 18]. Whether this increase in collagen is due to continued deposition of collagen with age or to the precipitation of soluble collagen or to both is not clearly defined. The pulpal stroma of non-erupted teeth consist of fine collagenous fibers interspersed in the ground substance. The conspicuous vascular and neural connective tissue sheaths are the only large collagen fiber bundles present; they fol-

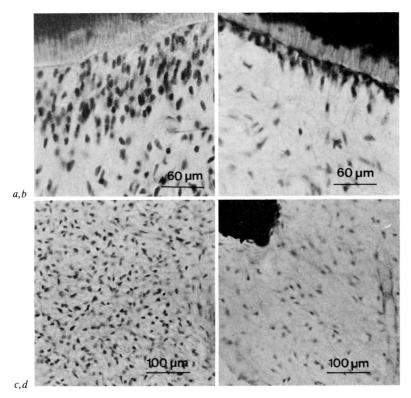

a,b

c,d

Fig. 4. a Section of the pulpo-odontoblastic area from an individual, 25 years old. The odontoblastic layer consists of seven or eight cell layers. ×150. *b* The pulpo-odontoblastic zone from 'old' tooth. Note the marked decrease in the number of odontoblasts. ×150. *c* The pulp proper from the tooth illustrated in *a*. There is a greater number of cells in the pulp than seen in the older pulp illustrated in figure 4d. ×75. *d* The pulp proper from the tooth illustrated in *b*. Note the sparsity of cells within the connective tissue stroma. ×75. All sections were stained with iron hematoxylin.

low the pathways of the nerves and blood vessels (fig. 5a, b). The orientation of the vascular and neural sheaths is further emphasized in sections of young functional pulps that are impregnated with silver nitrate or picrofuchsin. Figure 6 illustrates a silver nitrate-impregnated section of such a tooth. It is apparent that the large collagen fiber bundles are directly associated with the pathways of blood vessels and nerves. When the sections of young adult pulps are examined under higher magnification, the pulpal stroma still consist of fine collagenous fibers, and the only thick argyrophilic fiber bundles are the connective tissue sheaths of lost blood

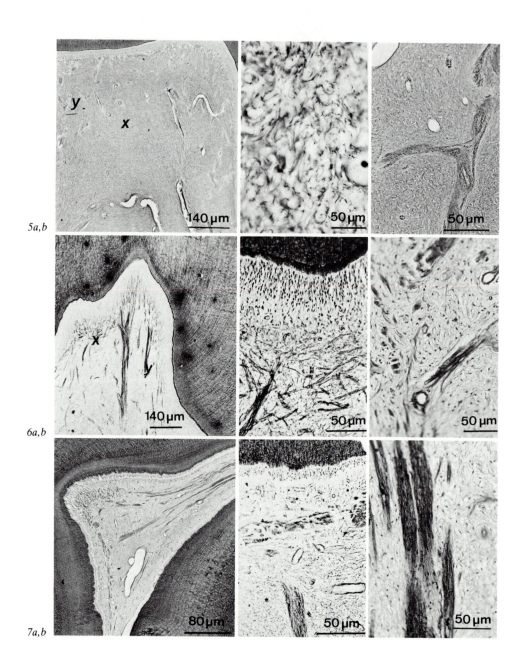

5a,b

6a,b

7a,b

vessels and nerves (fig. 6a, b). The prominence of the connective tissue sheaths is further accentuated in the 'old' pulps as seen in figure 7. In figure 7a, b, one observes small bundles of collagen fibers in which degenerated nerves were found. The fibrosis appears, therefore, to be related to the pathways of the degenerated vessels or nerves.

In summary, it can be said that the coronal pulps of old teeth show a relative increase in the number of thick collagenous bundles. These fibrous bundles are the connective tissue sheaths of degenerated blood vessels and nerves. The stroma of the pulp still consists of fine collagenous fibers. Changes as the result of aging in collagen in the skin and elsewhere have been summarized by Verzar [30], Gross [15] and Milch [12]. They all agree that there is an increase in the thickness of the collagen fibers and changes in the chemical and physical properties of the collagen during the aging process. The pulpal stroma, in contrast to the dermis of the skin, consists mainly of fine collagenous fibers interspersed in the abundant ground substance. At no time during the life of the tooth are thick collagen fibers seen independently of the connective tissue sheaths. The data of the current study indicate that the connective tissue of the pulp is specialized in nature; no comparison can be made between the effects of aging on the connective tissue of the pulp and those on other areas rich in connective tissue such as skin or even gingiva.

Our findings also agree with the conclusions of Shroff [27] and Stanley and Ranney [28] that pulpal fibrosis in old teeth is not the result of a continual formation and reorientation of collagen fibers during the aging process. The prominence of fiber bundles in old pulps may be, in part, attributed to the persistence of the connective tissue sheaths in a narrowed pulpal chamber after the vascular and neural structures are decreased or lost.

Fig. 5. Section from a non-erupted third molar tooth from a young adult 20 years of age. The sections were treated with silver nitrate impregnation for the demonstration of collagen fibers. Note that the pulp consists mainly of fine small collagen fibers. ×35. *a* High magnification of area X shows the fine small fibers. ×125. *b* High magnification of area Y shows that thick fiber bundles are associated with the blood vessels and nerves. ×125.

Fig. 6. Section of an adult functional tooth from a 30-year-old individual. Neural and vascular connective tissue sheaths are prominent ×35. *a* High magnification at the pulpo-odontoblastic region of pulp (area X). Note that the thick fiber bundles are neural or vascular connective tissue sheaths; the stroma is made up of fine argyrophilic fibers. *b* Higher magnification of area Y. Note that the collagen fiber bundles are neural sheaths. ×250.

Fig. 7. Section from an 'aged' tooth. Thick fiber bundles appear to follow the pathways of nerves and vessels. ×20. *a* High magnification of the pulpo-odontoblastic region. The thick fiber bundles are prominent and related to the pathways of old blood vessels and nerves. *b* The stroma still consists of fine small collagen fibers. Note the thick neural sheath of a nerve. ×250.

Von Korff Fibers

During the aging process, the Von Korff fibers (collagenous fibers that emerge from the predentine and pass into the pulp) become accentuated. In unerupted teeth, fine Von Korff fibers emerge from the predentine to pass through the odontoblastic layer into the zone of Weil (fig. 8a). The argyrophilic fibers become more prominent with eruption and function, and extend into the pulpo-odontoblastic border (fig. 8b). The predentine-pulpal border in the old teeth was very irregular in outline. Concomitantly, there was a fusion of the fine Von Korff fibers. These fibers appear to form short bundles that are limited in their course to the odontoblastic layer (fig. 8c).

Changes in Ground Substance

The semiqualitative presence of the protein-acid mucopolysaccharide (GAG) complex is demonstrated by the Alcian blue-PAS combination. With this histochemical reaction, the GAG are alcianophilic whereas the glycoproteins and sialic acid are Schiff-positive. When sections of young functional, and old teeth, respectively, are exposed to this histochemical combination, the predentine and the pulp are Alcian blue-positive whereas the dentine stains pink in the young pulps. There is little difference in the intensity of alcianophilia between the young and old pulps. The coronal and root pulpal tissue is Alcian blue-positive. The core of the root and crown pulp is alcianophilic in old pulps. The presence of the calcified masses in the root pulp accentuates the Schiff intensity, becoming deep red in color. When there is diffuse calcification in the coronal pulp, the calcified masses stain Schiff-positive in contrast to the surrounding pulpal ground substance which appears deep blue (fig. 9).

Since the pulp is of loose connective tissue in nature, it is rich in proteoglycans. It thus stains intensely blue with Alcian blue. The staining response of the pulp of old teeth to the Alcian blue and PAS combination do not change drastically from that in the young pulps. The only structures that react differently with this histochemical combination are the vascular and neural connective tissue sheaths. In contrast to the alcianophilia of these collagen bundles in young pulps, the old fibrous bundles are Schiff-positive. Bhussrey [8] and Zerlotti [32] reported a decrease in mucopolysaccharides in aging pulps, and Mancini et al. [21], Wentz et al. [31] and Larincz [20 agreed that the amount of amorphous ground substances decreases as the number of collagen fibrils increases in the skin and elsewhere. Since we did not carry out any biochemical analy-

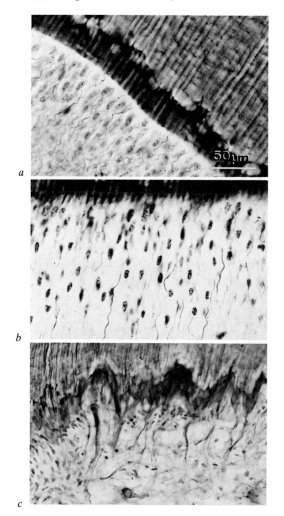

Fig. 8. a Odontoblastic-predentine region from a non-erupted molar tooth. Note fine collagenous fiber (Von Korffs) emerging from the predentine and passing into Zone of Weil. Silver nitrate impregnation. ×125. *b* Young adult tooth. The collagenous fibers are thicker and pass through the Zone of Weil into pulp proper. ×125. *c* An aged tooth. In contrast to long individual fibers seen in preceding illustration, fibers in the old tooth appear to fuse into short, thick fiber bundles that terminate in the Zone of Weil. ×125. All sections were exposed to silver nitrate impregnation.

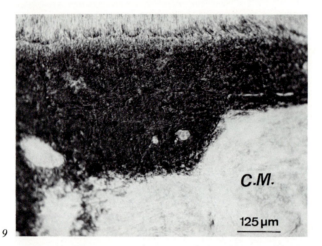

9

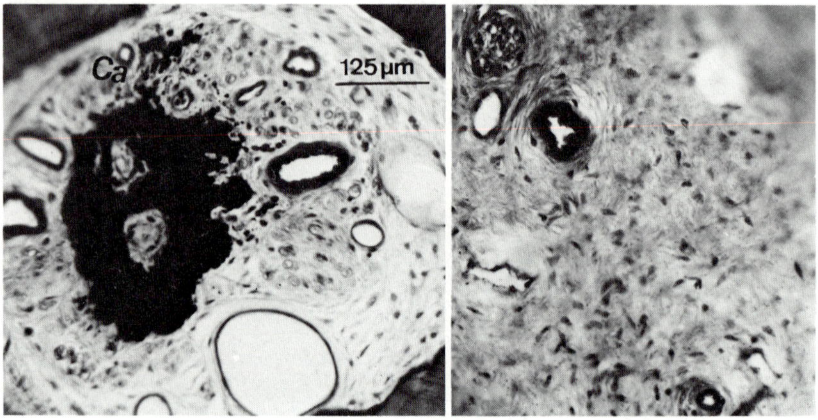

10a,b

Fig. 9. Section of a molar tooth from an individual over 55 years of age. The section was exposed to Alcian blue (pH 2.5) – PAS combination. The dystrophic calcified mass (CM) stained red while the remaining connective tissue stroma appeared Alcian blue-positive. ×125.

Fig. 10. a Cross-sectional view of the root pulp of a first molar from an 'aged' individual. The cross-sectional area of the pulp is reduced by the continual deposition of dentine. Notice the nerves and vessels concentrated in the core of the pulp, and the presence of diffuse calcified masses. The walls of the arterioles, venules, and capillaries are strongly PAS-positive. PAS-hematoxylin. Ca., capillary. ×125. *b* A cross-sectional view of the root pulp from a young adult. Note the mesenchymal-like tissue that makes up the core of the pulp, and the arterioles, venules and nerves. PAS-hematoxylin. ×125.

sis no definite conclusion can be drawn as to the amount and nature of the mucopolysaccharide-protein complex in old pulps. However, the semi-qualitative histochemical data from the study by Bernick and Nedelman [5] would indicate that any comparison with the loss of ground substance in skin and other connective tissue areas is not valid because the nature and amount of mucopolysaccharides differ in each tissue. In addition, it may be assumed that the decrease in ground substance previously reported for old pulps may be partly due to the decrease in the pulpal area and not to the nature of the carbohydrate moiety.

Vascular and Nerve Distribution

Aging leads to degenerative changes to vascular and nerve supply to the pulp. In the root pulps of old teeth there is a narrowing of the circumference. The blood vessels and nerves are aggregated in the core of the pulp and appear very prominent (fig. 10a). The small arteries and veins appear intensely red following staining with PAS. A large dystrophic calcification is observed in the above figure. On the other hand a cross-sectional view of the root pulp from a 'young' tooth reveals a mesenchyme-like tissue that forms the stroma of the pulp, and the arteries, veins, and nerves are located throughout the pulp (fig. 10b).

One of the first alterations to be observed to the small arteries in the root pulp in aging teeth is arteriosclerotic changes. Figure 11a illustrates such a small artery. The intima of the vessel is thickened resulting in a small lumen. No such changes are demonstrable in the arteries of pulps from the younger teeth (fig. 11b). The walls of the arterioles in the pulps from the old teeth appeared intensely red following the PAS reaction (fig. 12a). This positive reaction was not obtained when the arterioles from young teeth were exposed to the same staining reaction (fig. 12b). The old blood capillaries exhibited a widening of the basement membranes with strongly PAS-positive staining whereas the young vessels appeared to have thin lightly red-stained membranes (fig. 10a, 13d).

In the process of diffuse calcification of the root pulp the adventitia and media of the small arteries, and veins as well as the walls of capillaries become mineralized, eventually leading to the loss of vessels in the old pulps (fig. 13a–d). With the continual apposition of dentine and diffuse calcified masses, the circumference and area of the pulp decrease.

This leads to closure of the apical foramen with only one blood vessel entering the root pulp (fig. 14). In the coronal pulp from teeth obtained from individuals under 45 years of age, the arteries and veins enter the coronal pulp where they branch extensively both laterally and occusally

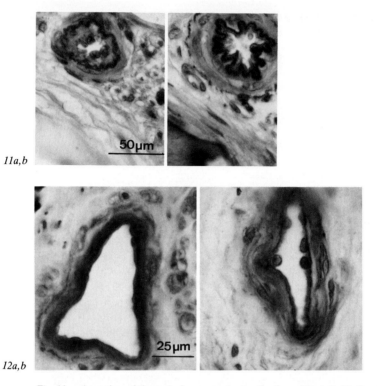

11a,b

12a,b

Fig. 11. a A section of the pulp from a molar tooth of an old adult. Notice the typical intimal hyperplasia characterized by proliferation of cells, collagenous and elastic fibers. Verhoeff's iron hematoxylin. ×350. *b* A section of the pulp from a molar tooth from a young adult. In contrast to the vessel seen in *a*, the intima of this vessel consists mainly of an endothelial cell abutting against the internal elastic fibers. Verhoeff's iron hematoxylin. ×350.

Fig. 12. a A cross-section of a typical arteriole in the pulp of first molar from an old adult. Notice the thick PAS-positive staining of the wall of this vessel. PAS-hematoxylin. ×500. *b* A cross-section of a typical arteriole in the pulp of first molar from a 'young' tooth. The wall of this vessel appears light red in color. The internal elastic lamina stains positive with PAS. PAS-hematoxylin. ×500.

to reach the zone of Weil where they form a subodontoblastic plexus (fig. 15a). From the plexus arterioles venules and capillaries enter the odontoblastic layer to form a layer of capillaries lined up adjacent to the predentine (fig. 15b). The sparsity of the blood vascular elements in the aged coronal pulp of a 63-year-old male is illustrated in figure 16a. The pulp exhibits an apparent increase in collagenous fibers and calcified masses. Cuspal vessels that persist are calcified along their walls. There is also a marked loss of terminal capillaries in the subodontoblastic layer (fig. 16b).

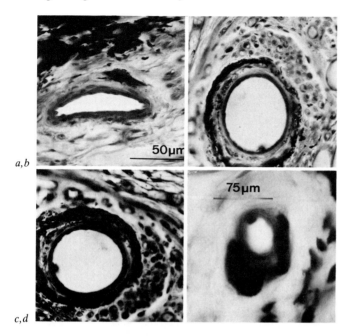

a,b

c,d

Fig. 13. a A section of a premolar from an old adult. Note the presence of a calcified mass at the edge of the adventitia of the arteriole. ×400. *b* A section of an arteriole found in the pulp of a molar tooth from an old adult. Note the circumferential calcification of the adventitia, the beginning mineralization in the media, and the thick PAS-positive basement membrane underneath the endothelial layer. ×400. *c* A section of an arteriole in the pulp of a molar tooth from a 70-year-old male. Note the extensive calcification of all the layers of the vessel. ×400. *d* A section of a capillary found in the pulp of a molar tooth from the 70-year-old male *(c)*. Note the thickened basement membrane, and the calcification around it. ×600. All the sections were exposed to the PAS-hematoxylin.

The lymphatic capillaries and collecting vessels in old teeth do not show changes following the PAS reaction as they are not encircled by an intact basement membrane. Figure 17 illustrates an aged molar tooth, containing diffuse calcified masses in its pulp. In addition the tooth is carious. Under higher magnification lymphatic collecting vessels appear dilated among inflammatory cells (fig. 17a).

As with the blood vascular system, the nerves within the root pulp exhibited changes as result of the diffuse calcification. The connective tissue sheaths of the nerve bundles become mineralized (fig. 18a). The mineralizing process was progressive in nature and soon adjacent nerve bundles were completely obliterated as seen in figure 18b, c. There is

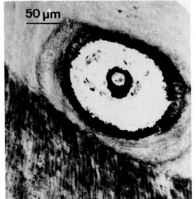

14

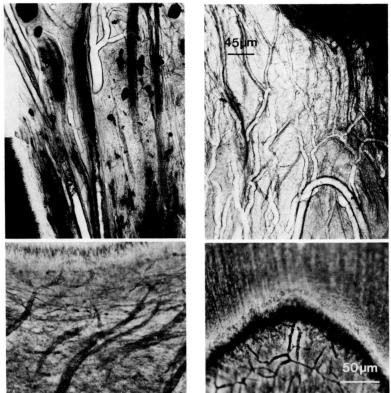

15a,b

16a,b

extensive branching of nerves in the coronal pulp from young and mature teeth. The pulpal nerves when they reach the cuspal zone form a sub-odontoblastic plexus (fig. 19). From this plexus non-medullated nerves enter the odontoblastic layer to terminate among the odontoblasts (fig. 19a). The paucity of nerves in old pulps is seen in figure 20a, a section of a tooth from a 60-year-old person. Cuspal nerves and their terminal branching are absent (fig. 20b). The nerve fibers that persist show signs of degeneration such as reticulation, fragmentation, and beading (fig. 20c).

The preservation of the structural integrity of the pulp is the function of the blood lymphatic vascular system as well as the connective tissue interstitium. In the young adult pulp the essential substances are transferred from the blood capillaries to the loose connective tissue interstitium and to the odontoblasts. The metabolic byproducts must be returned to the blood in the same manner. Accumulation of extracellular interstitial material not returned directly by the blood system is removed by the lymphatic vessels before returning to the blood vascular system [1, 10, 13].

The finding of thick-walled blood capillaries in the aging pulps is similar to what has been described in the aging gingivae [6], periodontal ligament [14] and tongue [11]. The importance of the thickened capillary basement membrane in the aged human pulp is as a potential barrier to exchange of smaller molecules. Bastal [2] and Reis [25] demonstrated that capillary permeability decreases with age. In addition, Jones [19] described a substantial decrease in the exchange of O_2 and CO_2 with age in man. Thus, transfer of substances from blood to cells may be slowed during aging. This process may be reflected in a decrease in the number of cells in the aged pulp.

Fig. 14. A section of the apical portion of the pulp from an incisor tooth obtained from a 68-year-old female. Continuous deposition of both dentine and diffuse calcification has resulted in narrowing of the pulpal circumference so that only one vessel is demonstrable. The vessel is also circumscribed by a calcified ring. PAS-hematoxylin. ×250.

Fig. 15. a A thick section of the coronal portion of the pulp of a premolar tooth from a young adult. Note the dense vascular network coursing throughout the pulp. Iron hematoxylin. ×125. b A section of the cuspal ara of the pulp of a young adult molar. The capillaries have penetrated the odontoblastic zone to abut against the predentine. Iron hematoxylin. ×125.

Fig. 16. a A thick section (150) of the coronal portion of the pulp of a premolar from an old adult. Note (1) diffuse calcification throughout the crown of the pulp, (2) the calcified blood vessels, (3) the loss of demonstrable vessels throughout the pulp. Iron hematoxylin. ×50. b A section of the occlusal area of the pulp from an 'old' tooth. Note the loss of capillary network within the odontoblastic layer. ×50.

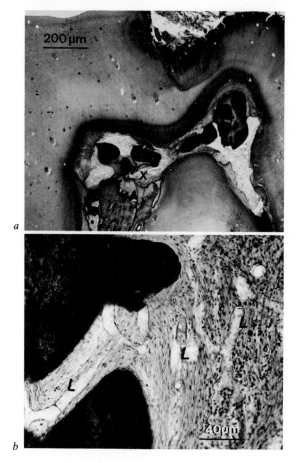

Fig. 17. a Section of an 'old' tooth that shows a marked deposition of dystrophic calcification as well as of a carious invasion into the pulp. PAS-hematoxylin. ×50. *b* Higher
magnification of area 'X'. Note the pulpal inflammatory cells. The lymphatic collecting vessels within the inflammatory area appear dilated. L = Lymphatic collecting vessel. ×100.

The absence of an intact basement membrane around the lymphatic
capillaries, and the type of endothelial cell junctions provide an uninter-
rupted passage of fluid from the interstitium into lymphatic vessels. Since
no structural change in lymphatic vessels have been described with the
light microscopy in the pulps of aged humans, the removal of water, elec-
trolytes, and macromolecules by this route has probably not altered.

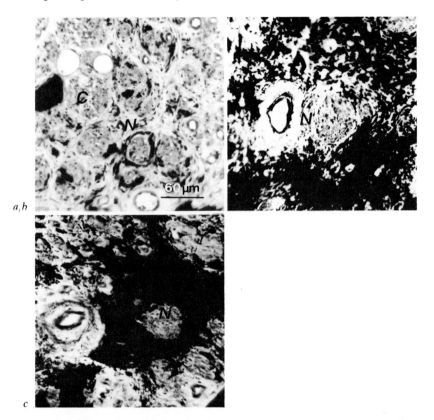

Fig. 18. a Cross-sectional view of the root pulp of a premolar from a 50-year-old individual. There are isolated regions of calcification in the perineurium and endoneurium of nerve fasciculi and individual fibers. N = Nerve. ×150. *b* Cross-sectional view of root pulp from a molar from a 60-year-old individual. Note the progressive calcification of the pulp obliterating nerve fibers. ×150. *c* Cross-sectional view of root from a molar from a 60-year-old individual. The calcified mass has obliterated all but two nerve fibers. ×150. All sections were stained with iron hematoxylin.

The blood and lymphatic microvasculature play an important role in the early phases of inflammation, increased blood content, increased capillary and venule permeability, and the migration of blood cells to the area of injury. The clearance of excessive fluid, proteins, macromolecules, and cells which accumulate within the interstitium in an inflamed area is provided by the lymphatic vascular system. There is no available data in the literature regarding microvascular aging in early pulpal inflammation. However, it could be theorized that the altered chemical and physical properties of the thickened PAS-positive adventitia of

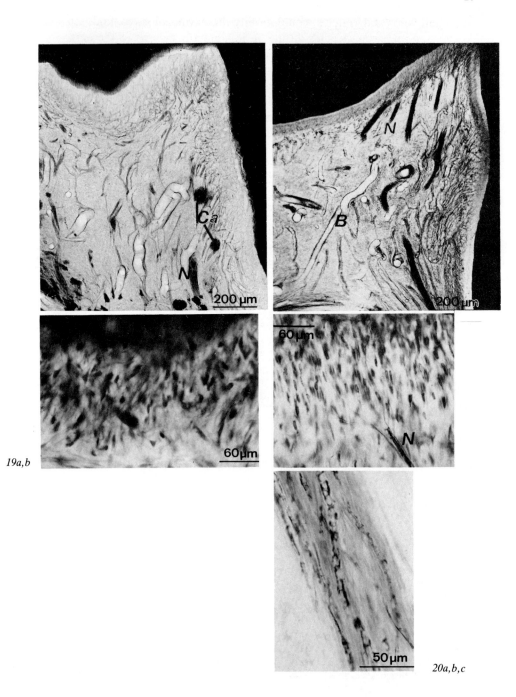

19a,b

20a,b,c

the small veins and venules, could modify the permeability to fluid, leukocytes and macromolecules during an inflammatory insult to the aging pulp. This would delay the resolution of a carious invasion into the pulp. On the other hand, the lymphatic capillaries are still untouched by the aging process, so that they would be able to provide sufficient drainage for the removal of inflammatory cells, fluid and particulate from the injured aged pulp depending upon the severity of the inflammatory process.

Conclusions

The age related changes to the human dental pulp as described in the present report can be summarized as follows: (1) pulp volume decreases progressively from the eruption of the tooth to 'old' age; (2) dystrophic calcification occurs in both the root and coronal pulp; (3) the number of cells, collagen fibers, and ground substance alters; (4) blood vessels and nerves are lost. These changes demonstrable in the pulps or old teeth resemble those reported in other connective tissues of the body [9, 15, 22, 30]. All agree that changes take place in the physical and chemical properties of collagen. There is an increase in the tensile strength of the collagen fibrils, together with a loss of extensibility and an increase in thermal contraction. Old collagen has been known to resist proteolytic enzyme action. A decrease in the ratio of chondroitin sulfate to hyaluronic acid has been noted in the ground substance of tongue and gingivae in humans of advancing age [22].

The diffuse calcification seen in the pulps of teeth from individuals over the age of 50 years could have been predicted from the changes to the collagen fibers. Milch [22] postulated that an apparent increase in the cross-linkage of collagen with advancing age enhances its tendency for calcification. Collagen fibers forming the neural sheaths and the adventi-

---

Fig. 19. a A thick section of the coronal portion of the pulp from a molar tooth from a 'teenage' individual. Pulpal nerve divides into cuspal nerves. Note that subodontoblastic network. N = Nerves; B = blood vessels. ×50. *b* A higher magnification of the subodontoblastic plexus. Nerves from this network pass into the odontoblastic zone. ×150.

Fig. 20. a A thick section of the coronal pulp from a 65-year-old male. Note that the pulp contain loci of calcification and increased fibrosis. There is an apparent decrease in the number of nerves in the pulp proper and in the subodontoblastic area. ×50. *b* A higher magnification of area 'X'. Note that absence of nerves in the odontoblastic zone. ×150. *c* A high magnification of a nerve in the pulp illustrated in figure 20a. Note the fragmentation, beading and reticulation of the nerve fiber characteristic of a degenerating nerve. ×450.

tia of blood vessels in the old pulps stain deep red with the PAS reaction, a response not seen in 'young' collagen. The intense Schiff-positive collagen fibers become the loci for calcification in an environment that is potentially a calcifying medium. Another example supporting this thesis is the calcification of the attachment fibers in 'old' human periodontal ligament [14], another potential calcification site.

The progressive dystrophic calcification begins in the root pulp and extends into the coronal pulp. Further deposition of calcified tissue may lead to the obliteration of pulpal tissue in the root and coronal pulps. In addition the calcification of the connective tissue sheaths of the nerves and blood vessels leads to the loss of both nerves and blood vessels of different caliber in the root and crown of old teeth. The deviations from the nerve and vascular patterns seen in the 'young' pulps might help explain the decrease in sensitivity and metabolic rate of the pulps in 'aged' persons. The loss of vessels forming the microvasculature as well as changes in the remaining arterioles, capillaries, and venules would lead to a decrease in the rate of transfer of nutrients from the blood stream to the interstitium and finally to the pulpal cells as well as the odontoblasts. This would bring about a decrease in the number of viable fibroblasts and odontoblasts. The dependency of the dentine on the pulp is well recognized. Changes in the pulpal elements are reflected in changes in the dentine. Alterations in the collagen fibers and ground substance in the dentine would increase calcification of peritubular dentine resulting in narrowing of the tubules as well as producing sclerosis.

Age changes in the pulp affect the response of pulpal elements to injury and repair. The alterations to the microvasculature would hinder both the hemodynamic and cellular responses in the resolution of inflammation within the pulp. The loss of fibroblasts and odontoblasts would impair the repair phase of healing.

An understanding of these morphological alterations that occur during the aging process is important, for such knowledge will help in the understanding of the functional age changes that may lead to decreased activity in the aged and predispose the aged individuals to pulpal disease or loss of teeth.

References

1 Allen, L.: Lymphatics and lympoid tissues. A. Rev. Physiol. *29:* 197–224 (1967).
2 Bastal, P.: Die abiologischen Grundlagen des Alterns. Z. Alternsforsch. *9:* 211–219 (1955).
3 Bernick, S.: Age changes in the blood supply to human teeth. J. dent. Res. *46:* 544–550 (1967).

4   Bernick, S.: Effect of aging on the nerve supply to human teeth. J. dent. Res. *46:* 694–699 (1967).

5   Bernick, S.; Nedelman, C.: Effect of aging on the human pulp. J. Endocr. *1:* 88–94 (1975).

6   Bernick, S.; Sobin, S.: The lymphatic and blood vessels of the aged human gingiva. Gerodontology *1:* 65–71 (1982).

7   Bernick, S.; Sobin, S.; Paule, W. J.: Changes in the microvasculature and interstitium of aged human mandibles and maxillae. Gerodontology *2:* 9–14 (1983).

8   Bhussery, B. R.: Modification of the dental pulp during development and aging; in Finn. Biology of the dental pulp, pp. 146–165 (University of Alabama Press, University of Alabama 1968).

9   Clausen, B.: Aging of connective tissue; in Asboe-Hansen, hormones and connective tissue. Williams and Wilkins, Co. (1966).

10 Courtice, C.: Lymph and plasma proteins: barrier to their movements throughout the extracellular fluid. Lymphology *4:* 9–17 (1971).

11 de Mignard, V. A.; Dreizen, S.; Bernick, S.: Aging changes in human tongue components. J. dent. Res. *60:* 545 (1981).

12 Frolich, E.: Altersveränderungen der Pulp und des Paradontium. Dt. zahnärztl. Z. *25:* 175–183 (1970).

13 Foldi, M.: Diseases of lymphatics and lymph circulation; 2nd ed. (Pergammon Press, Oxford 1967).

14 Grant, D. A.; Bernick, S.: The peridontium of aging humans. J. Perlodont. *4:* 660–667 (1972).

15 Gross, J. Aging of connective tissue; the extracellular components; in Bourne, Structural aspects of ageing, pp. 177–195 (Hafner, New York 1961).

16 Han, S. S.: The fine structure of cells and intercellular substance of the dental pulp; in Finn, Biology of the dental pulp organ, pp. 103–139 (University of Alabama Press, University of Alabama 1968).

17 Hill, T. J. Textbook of oral pathology, pp. 211–217 (Lea & Febiger, Philadelphia 1949).

18 Ingle, J. I. Etiology of pulp. Inflammation necrosis or dystrophy; in Ogilvie, Ingle, Atlas of pulp and periapical biology, p. 289 (Lea & Febiger, Philadelphia 1965).

19 Jones, H. B.: Molecular exchange and blood perfusion through tissue regions. Adv. biol. med. Phys. *2:* 53–77 (1971).

20 Larincz, A. L.: Physiology of the aging skin. III. Med. J. *117:* 59 (1960).

21 Mancini, R. E.; Vilar, O.; Stein, E.; Fiorini, H.: Histochemical study of postnatal development of skin connective tissue. Rev. Soc. Argent. Biol. *53:* 196 (1959).

22 Milch, R. A. S.: Aging of connective tissue; in Shock, pp. 109–124 (Thomas, Springfield 1966).

23 Pinzon, R. D.; Toto, P. D.; O'Malley, J. J.: Kinetics of rat molar pulp cells at various ages. J. dent. Res. *45:* 934–938 (1966).

24 Pinzon, R. D.; Kozlow, M.; Burch, W. P.: Histology of rat molar pulp at different ages. J. dent. Res. *46:* 202–208 (1967).

25 Reis, W.: Aging of the capillary system. Dt. Gesundhwes. *16:* 580–585 (1961).

26 Seltzer, S.; Bender, I. B.: Retrogressive and age changes of the dental pulp; in The dental pulp. Biologic considerations in dental procedures; 2nd ed., pp. 291–314 (Lippincot, Phildelphia 1975).

27 Shroff, F. R.: Physiologic pathology of changes in the dental pulp. Senile pulp atrophy. Oral Surg. *6:* 1,455–1,460 (1953).

28 Stanley, H. R.; Ranney, R. R.: Age changes in the human pulp. The quality of collagen. Oral Surg. *15:* 1,396–1,404 (1962).

29 Ten Cate, A. R.: Dental pulp complex; in Ten Cate, Oral histology, pp. 178–181 (Mosby, St. Louis 1980).
30 Verzar, F.: Ageing of collagen fibers; in Hall, International review of connective tissue, vol. 2, pp. 224–282 (Academic Press, New York 1964).
31 Wentz, F. W.; Maier, A. W.; Orban, B.: Age changes and sex differences in the clinically 'normal' gingiva. J. Periodont. 23: 12–24 (1952).
32 Zerlotti, E.: Histochemical study of the connective tissue of the dental pulp. Archs oral Biol. 9: 149–162 (1964).

Sol Bernick, PhD, Department of Anatomy and Cell Biology, University of Southern California, School of Medicine, Los Angeles, CA 90033 (USA)

Front. oral Physiol., vol. 6, pp. 31–39 (Karger, Basel 1987)

Morphological Changes in Human Salivary Glands

J. R. Drummond

Department of Dental Prosthetics and Gerontology, Dental School and Hospital, Dundee, Scotland

Introduction

Progressive age-related alterations in the morphology of the human major and minor salivary glands have been described and include fibrosis, adiposity and loss of acinar elements. Knowledge of these changes have been obtained predominantly from postmortem studies, although some studies of the minor glands have used volunteer patients.

Major Salivary Glands

Early studies of the human major salivary glands were descriptive or semiquantitative. Andrew [2], in 1952, published an account of age changes observed in the parotid and submandibular glands. In the parotid glands he considered that in extreme old age up to 50% of acinar elements may be replaced by adipose tissue. In submandibular glands adipose tissue was also noted in old age but in a lower proportion, fibrous tissue being more prominent. Andrew [2] also observed chronic inflammatory infiltrates throughout the submandibular and parotid glands. Increases in the large eosinophilic oncocytic cells, sometimes associated with ducts, were observed in a few glands. These cells, the function of which remains unknown, have been shown to contain a great many mitochondria in their cytoplasm [24]. Their association with salivary glands in senile individuals is therefore difficult to explain.

Waterhouse et al. [27] applied point counting to a series of 36 randomly selected submandibular glands obtained from postmortems. Six glands for each age decade from 25 to 85 years were studied and these showed a progressive replacement of functional cells by adipose tissue. In a few glands from the youngest age group some adipose cells were noted.

On average, between childhood and old age one quarter of functional cells may be lost and in extreme cases one half. Although the adiposity of the salivary glands was previously believed to be related to the general adiposity of the individual [25], the study of Waterhouse et al. [27] provides contrary evidence. No relationship could be found between the adiposity of individuals and the proportion of adipose tissue in the submandibular glands indicating, in these glands at least, that the glands do not behave as a functional part of the body's 'fat organ'.

Although adipose cells in salivary glands have previously been considered to be the end result of degenerative destruction of acinar elements there seems little evidence to support this view. Garrett [11] has noted intracellular fat droplets in serous acini, mucous acini and ducts but could see little evidence of droplet fusion which would indicate cellular degeneration. Furthermore, if the adipose cells are examined using stains for nerve tissue no nerve plexus is noted, although we would have expected to see this, if these cells had previously been acinar cells. The weight of evidence seems to suggest, therefore, that a replacement process is involved rather than a destructive process.

In a series of papers published between 1975 and 1980, Scott [13–20] has provided more detailed quantitative information on age changes in the submandibular glands. In a paper published in 1975 Scott [13] showed the relationship between age and submandibular gland volumes. Variation in gland volumes between individuals was wide, ranging from below 2 cm^3 to over 15 cm^3 and male glands were larger on average by 50%. In both male and female glands a reduction in mean volume in old age was noted although only in the female group was this statistically significant. Contralateral glands from the same individual also show considerable variation, the mean being 6.2% difference for males and 6.9% difference for females. In some glands there could be as much as a 28% difference while in only 7 individuals out of 75 was the contralateral difference insignificant (less than 1%). These variations between individuals and between right and left submandibular glands in the same individual have obvious implications when measurements are being made of submandibular salivary flow rates.

In a quantitative histological study of the submandibular glands Scott [15] has provided information on changes in volume proportion of various gland components in each of the age decades from 16 to 95 years. A summary of mean values for the youngest and oldest age decades is shown in table I. These results show that while the proportion volume of parenchyma is reduced with age, only the acini are in fact reduced and there is indeed an increase in ductal elements. In a further study Scott [19] has counted mucous and serous cells separately and concluded that

Table I. Mean proportion volumes ± SE in youngest and oldest age decades. From ref. [15]

	Parenchyma %	Acini %	Ducts %	Vascular tissue %	Adipose tissue %
Youngest decade (16–25 years)	70.45 ±1.29	62.03 ±1.50	8.42 ±0.37	4.56 ±0.36	4.27 ±0.99
Oldest decade (86–95 years)	49.16 ±1.73	43.43 ±1.59	10.64 ±0.55	7.28 ±0.57	15.05 ±1.47

although the proportion of mucous cells vary widely between individuals (mean 7.8%) no significant age or sex differences could be found. The increase in ductal elements can be accounted for by increases in non-striated and extralobular ducts. Two thirds of the increase in ductal volume can be accounted for by an increase in the non-striated intralobular ducts. Striated ducts although usually forming the largest proportion of the duct system remained static at about 5% of total gland volume.

Qualitative changes can also be observed in the various components of the submandibular glands in the elderly. With increasing age acini become less uniform in size and shape. Many acini are shrunken and others appear almost duct-like with wide lumen [16]. The intralobular ducts show increasing dilation and hyperplasia with increasing age. Consolidated deposits of predominantly eosinophilic material are also noted in the small ducts and those also increase with age [18].

It will be noted in table I that the volume proportion of salivary blood vessels increase with age and deteriorative structural changes can also be observed. The changes observed are, increasing intimal and medial fibroelastosis, occasional medial calcification and infrequently atheroma. The senile changes noted in the vasculature and resultant changes in salivary gland blood flow may obviously be of importance, not only explaining parenchymal damage, but also changes in the quality and quantity of saliva secreted.

Thus far, no mention has been made of inflammatory changes found in the major salivary glands unaffected by disease. Two distinct types of inflammatory processes have been described in the submandibular glands [14]. Firstly, focal lymphocytic adenitis was defined as a collection of not less than 50 lymphocytes and plasma cells usually found surrounding small infralobular and interlobular ducts or blood vessels. The second type of inflammatory change, focal obstructive adenitis, consists of diffuse chronic inflammatory infiltration, fibrosis and loss of acini. Focal lymphocytic adenitis can be observed in nearly all submandibular glands and is not related to the age or sex of the subject [14, 26]. In contrast, focal obstructive adenitis, although found in the majority of glands, shows a marked increase with age [14]. A good correlation also exists between the severity of focal obstructive adenitis and the degree of fibrosis occurring in individual glands. The study of Scott [14] also provides good epidemiological evidence that the two inflammatory responses are distinct. Firstly, the age profiles of the two processes are different and the severity of the two processes in individual glands seems uncorrelated. Secondly, despite both changes being common, coincidence of both types in the same area of a gland is infrequent.

The reasons for the increase in focal obstructive adenitis with age are not clear. It is possibly related to repeated subclinical episodes of obstruction occurring sporadically throughout life. This obstruction could be caused by pressure on a duct, even possibly from infiltrating adipose tissue. Another suggestion is that the inflammatory deposits described by Scott [16] cause intraluminal obstruction and stagnation distal to this. Scott's [17] study of these intraluminal deposits, however, shows that although the deposits and incidence of focal obstructive adenitis both increase will age, when the effect of age is eliminated there is no correlation between them.

Minor Salivary Glands

It is only comparatively recently that detailed descriptions of the minor salivary glands have been published [7, 20]. Minor salivary glands are more readily accessible and are also of considerable clinical significance in the diagnosis of the salivary gland manifestations of the connective tissue disorders [3].

The labial salivary glands, which are exclusively mucous, show progressive fibrosis with age and show little tendency to increased adiposity. In young individuals the glands are divided into small lobules separated by thin connective tissue septa but in the elderly, lobules may be separated by thick fibrous bands. Acini may also be separated by fibrous tissue bands and may appear shrunken and poorly staining. In extreme cases whole glands may be replaced by fibrous tissue with no acini remaining. Ducts seem unaffected although some show dilation and hyperplasia. Mean percentage volumes for the various glands' constituents in the labial glands are shown in table II. Occasionally oncocytes are also observed in the labial glands of older individuals [7].

Table II. Mean proportion volumes ± SE in labial salivary glands. From ref. [7]

Age years	Acini 1%	Ducts 1%	Connective tissue %	Vascular tissue %
24–44	56.1 ±2.4	9.2 ±0.6	29.8 ±2.8	3.5 ±0.3
45–65	50.6 ±1.9	12.5 ±1.5	32.0 ±1.3	3.0 ±0.2
66+	36.8 ±1.6	13.5 ±1.3	44.5 ±1.0	3.8 ±0.2

Table III. Patient biopsy results – mean proportion volumes ± SE. From ref. [8]

	Acini %	Ducts %	Connective tissue %	Vascular tissue %
Rheumatoid arthritis (mean age 56 years)	40.5 ±1.6	11.3 ±0.7	43.09 ±1.4	3.0 ±0.1
Rheumatoid arthritis plus Sjögren's syndrome	27.0 ±1.7	13.2 ±0.6	55.1 ±1.6	3.5 ±0.2

Focal obstructive adenitis may be found in the labial salivary glands and the severity of this increases with age. Focal lymphocytic adenitis probably does not normally occur in the labial glands [4, 7], although some papers report the occasional normal gland with infiltrates [20, 22]. The diagnostic significance of the labial glands is that they are readily available and in a number of connective tissue disorders, particularly Sjögren's syndrome, show a high density of focal lymphocytic infiltrates [3, 6]. The labial glands in individuals with a connective tissue disorder may also show acinar atrophy. In an attempt to see if labial acinar atrophy is greater in patients with Sjögren's syndrome than with aged-matched controls, Drummond and Chisholm [8] conducted a quantitative histological study. Eighteen patients with Sjögren's syndrome and 18 with rheumatoid arthritis alone were compared with normal controlled patients through a range of ages. The results show that there is a greater loss of acini in both patient groups than would be expected as a result of age alone. Acinar loss was, however, significantly greater in the Sjögren's

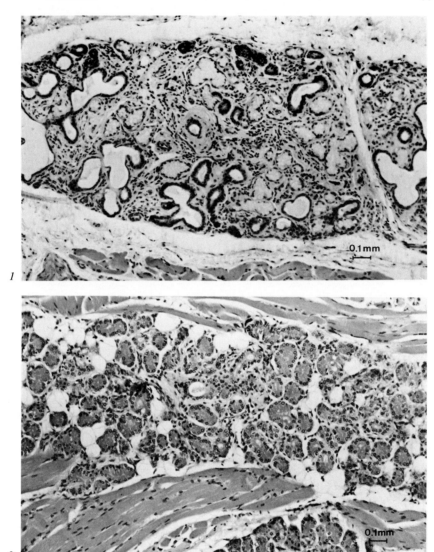

Fig. 1. Low-power view of a mucous lingual salivary gland from an elderly individual. Extensive acinar loss and fibrosis is seen along with a diffuse chronic inflammatory infiltrate. Ductal dilation is also shown.

Fig. 2. A serous lingual gland from a middle-aged individual which already shows adipose replacement of acinar elements.

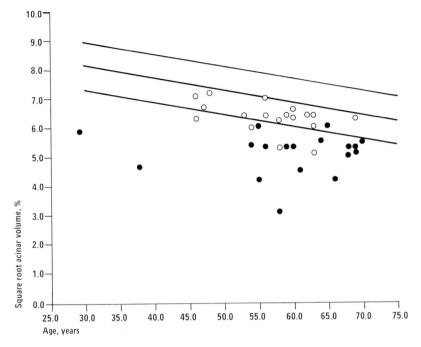

Fig. 3. Age-related loss in acinar volume proportion in the labial salivary glands with the 95% confidence limits marked. Individual Sjögren's syndrome results (●) show more extensive acinar loss than would be expected as a result of age alone. Rheumatoid arthritis patients (○) also show a greater loss although it is less dramatic.

syndrome patients than the rheumatoid arthritis patients alone (table III, fig. 1). The pathogenesis of the immunological destruction of salivary gland material in the connective tissues is not yet clear [1, 5, 6] although recently, using acid-α-naphthylacetate/esterase technique (ANAE), Syrjänen [22] has shown that the infiltrates in these glands are predominantly B lymphocytes. The mechanism of acinar loss in the aging process is also unclear and although B lymphocytes again predominate in the diffuse infiltrates it seems unlikely that identical mechanisms are involved. It would seem more likely that specific immunological processes take place in the salivary glands of Sjögren's syndrome patients already variably effected by an age-related acinar loss mediated by a different mechanism.

A detailed study of the lingual minor salivary glands removed from forensic postmortem subjects have also been undertaken [Drummond, 10]. One hundred and twenty tongues representative of age and sex from 20 to 80 years were used and salivary material examined from the posterior dorsum of the tongue. Both mucous and serous salivary glands are found in this area, and both show evidence of atrophic changes in old age. The mucous glands show changes very similar to those reported for the labial glands (fig. 2) while the serous glands show adipose replacement (fig. 3). Mast cell counts have also been carried out in the lingual glands [Drummond and McDiarmid, 9] and although there is no simple relationship with mast cell density and age some very fibrosed glands have high mast cell counts. Similar results have been recorded for the labial salivary glands Syrjänen and Syrjänen [23].

Concluding Remarks

Although extensive investigations have been made of the aging human salivary glands much work still needs to be undertaken. In particular studies at an electron microscope level should be undertaken and an extensive postmortem study of age changes in the parotid gland is required. Changes in the minor glands are of particular interest as alterations in their secretions in old age may have important clinical implications bearing in mind the unique properties of the saliva [12, 21]. More fundamental investigations should also be undertaken and monoclonal antibodies should be used to specifically identify inflammatory cells in senile glands. This, along with the development of a suitable animal model, may help to elucidate the underlying mechanisms involved which would have significant biological implications.

References

1   Anderson, L. G.; Tarpley, T. M.; Talal, N.; Cummings, N. A.; Wolf, R. O.; Schall, G. L.: Cellular – versus – humoral autoimmune response to salivary gland in Sjögren's syndrome. Clin. exp. Immunol. *13:* 335–339 (1973).
2   Andrew, W.: A comparison of age changes in the salivary glands of man and the rat. J. Geront. *7:* 178–182 (1952).
3   Chisholm, D. M.; Mason, D. K.: Labial salivary gland biopsy in Sjögren's syndrome. J. clin. Path. *21:* 656–700 (1968).
4   Chisholm, D. M.; Waterhouse, J. P.; Mason, D. K.: Lymphocytic sialadenitis in major and minor glands: a correlation in post-mortem subjects. J. clin. Path. *23:* 690–694 (1970).
5   Chused, T. M.; Hardin, J. A.; Frank, M. M.; Green, I.: Identification of cells infiltrating the minor salivary glands in patients with Sjögren's syndrome. J. Immun. *112:* 641–645 (1974).
6   Daniels, T. E.: Labial salivary gland biopsy in Sjögren's syndrome. Arthritis Rheum. *27:* 147–156 (1984).

7 Drummond, J. R.; Chisholm, D. M.: A qualitative and quantitative study of the human labial salivary glands. *29:* 151–155 (1984).

8 Drummond, J. R.; Chisholm, D. M.: A quantitative histological study of the human labial salivary glands in Sjögren's syndrome patients with and without rheumatoid arthritis. IRCS Med. Sci. vol. 14, pp. 118–119 (1986).

9 Drummond, J. R.; McDiarmid, M.: Mast cells in the human lingual salivary glands. J. dent. Res. vol. 65, p. 503 (1986).

10 Drummond, J. R.: The histology of the human lingual salivary glands. IRCS Med. Sci. Vol. 14, pp. 116–117 (1986).

11 Garrett, J. R.: Some observations on human submandibular salivary glands. Proc. R. Soc. Med. *55:* 488–491 (1962).

12 Green, D. R. G.; Embury, G.: The chemistry and biological properties of the minor salivary gland secretions; in Leach, Ericson, Oral interfacial reactions of bone, soft tissue and saliva Glantz, (IRL Press, 1985).

13 Scott, J.: Age, sex and contralateral differences in the volumes of human submandibular salivary glands. Archs. oral Biol. *20:* 885–887 (1975).

14 Scott, J.: The incidence of focal chronic inflammatory changes in human submandibular salivary glands. J. oral Pathol. *5:* 334–346 (1976).

15 Scott, J.: Quantitative age changes in the histological structure of the human submandibular salivary glands. Archs Oral Biol. *22:* 221–227 (1977).

16 Scott, J.: Degenerative changes in the histology of the human submandibular salivary glands occurring with age. J. Biol. buccale *5:* 311–319 (1977).

17 Scott, J.: A morphometric study of age changes in the histology of the ducts of the human submandibular salivary glands. Archs oral Biol. *22:* 243–249 (1977).

18 Scott, J.: The prevalence of consolidated salivary deposits in the small ducts of human submandibular glands. J. oral Pathol. *7:* 28–33 (1978).

19 Scott, J.: The proportional volume of mucous acinar cells in normal human submandibular salivary glands. Archs oral Biol. *24:* 479–481 (1979).

20 Scott, J.: Qualitative and quantitative observations on the histology of the human labial salivary glands obtained at post-mortem. J. Biol. buccale *8:* 182–200 (1980).

21 Slomiany, B. L.; Zdebska, E.; Murty, V. L. N.; Slomiany, A.; Petropoulou, K.; Mandel, I. D.: Lipid composition of human labial salivary gland secretions. Archs oral Biol. *28:* 711–714 (1983).

22 Syrjänen, S.: Salivary glands in rheumatoid arthritis; academic diss., Kuopio (1982).

23 Syrjänen, S. M.; Syrjänen, K. T.: Inflammatory cell infiltrate in labial salivary glands of patients with rheumatoid arthritis with special emphasis on tissue mast cells. Scand. J. dent. Res. *92:* 557–563 (1984).

24 Tandler, B.; Denning, C. R.; Mandel, I. D.; Kutscher, A. H.: Ultrastructure of the human labial salivary glands. III. Myoepithelilium and ducts. J. Morph. *130:* 227–233 (1970).

25 Wassermann, F.: The development of adipose tissue; in Renold, Cahill, Handbook of physiology, section 5, pp. 95–96 Am. Physiol. Soc., Washington.

26 Waterhouse, J. P.; Doniach, I.: Post-mortem prevalence of focal lymphocytic adenitis of the submandibular salivary gland. J. Path. Bact. *91:* 53–64 (1966).

27 Waterhouse, J. P.; Chisholm, D. M.; Winter, R. B.; Patel, M.; Yale, R. S.: Replacement of functional parenchymal cells by fat and connective tissue in human submandibular glands: an age-related change. J. oral Pathol. *2:* 16–27 (1973).

MR. J. R. Drummond, Department of Dental Prosthetics and Gerontology, Dental School and Hospital, Dundee DD1 4HN (Scotland)

Front. oral Physiol., vol. 6, pp. 40–62 (Karger, Basel 1987)

Structural Age Changes in Salivary Glands

John Scott

School of Dental Surgery, The University of Liverpool, Liverpool, England

Introduction

There is no doubt that salivary glands undergo histological changes with age. However, the predominant type of change encountered and the severity of the morphological disturbances sustained vary between species and between different types of glands. Much of the evidence for structural salivary age changes has come from observations on the major glands of man and the rat and it is evident from these studies that generalisations in regard to salivary aging may not always be appropriate. Certainly the morphological studies to date do not suggest a unified system of aging deterioration consistent for all types of salivary glands and all species.

Early descriptive accounts of age-related alterations of salivary structure in man and animals focused on atrophic changes in parenchymal components together with increasing fibrosis and adiposity [1–3, 16, 38]. More recently, with the application of stereological analysis to research in histopathology, it has been possible to confirm and extend many of these subjective findings by careful quantitative measurements.

These recent quantitative studies have provided a means to analyse the development of aging changes over the entire adult life span and have facilitated comparisons of their rates and extent between different glands. Importantly, they have also provided at least partial explanations for the seemingly different susceptibilities to functional impairments with age exhibited by the different salivary gland types [Baum, this volume]. However, before recounting the quantitative effects of aging it is necessary to describe the altered histological appearances which occur in many salivary glands between young and old adult life.

Qualitative Age Changes in Salivary Structure

Figure 1 provides a comparison of the different histology between young adult and old human submandibular glands. Their appearances are markedly different. The compact uniform parenchyma (acini plus ducts) which characterises the young-adult gland is replaced in old age by more loosely structured tissues in which the fibro-adipose supporting elements are more abundant, the ducts are dilated and more numerous, and the acini are more widely spaced and variable in size, shape and staining capacity. Broadly similar changes occur in other human salivary glands, e.g. parotid and labial. However, these differences are less representative of the changes developing in the rat salivary glands with age. The following sections deal with the various histological features in detail.

Parenchymal Changes

Depending on the species and the type of gland, the salivary parenchyma consists of serous, mucous or mixed acini together with various types of ducts arranged into morphological units of lobules which in turn are grouped into lobes. In human glands there is a progressive disparity of size and shape of lobes and lobules as age increases. Furthermore, as originally described by Hamperl [16] in 1931, there is evidence of age-related atrophy of acini and a relative increase in the intralobular ducts.

In man, the acini may exhibit loss of granules and cell shrinkage with age so that their lumens become wider and they resemble primitive ducts (fig. 2), while the intralobular ducts themselves become hyperplastic and dilated [16, 26]. Dilatation is also a feature of the extralobular ducts in old age. More rarely, these larger ducts may also exhibit basal metaplasia and hyperplasia with occasional obliteration of the lumens [26].

Ductal dilatation within the lobules is particularly a feature of aging human minor salivary glands [11, 12, 31] among which the labial glands have been most extensively studied. In old age they often show severe acinar atrophy in addition to the ductal changes of dilatation and hyperplasia (fig. 3). However, both the duct dilatation and loss of acini in these superficially exposed glands may be as much a product of repeated minor trauma and partial obstruction as an inherent feature of the aging processes alone. Similar age changes develop in the palatal and lingual glands although usually not so severely as in the labial glands.

In the salivary glands of laboratory animals, e.g. the rat, the gross parenchymal age changes appear less severe than those seen in man [19, 32]. Changes at a subcellular level, on the other hand, have been better categorised than in human glands.

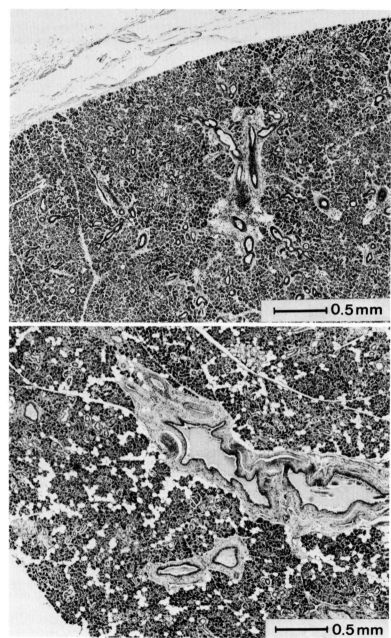

1a,b

Rats have been designated 'old' at various ages, usually from 700 days onwards. In such rats changes in the morphology of the nucleus of acinar cells are characteristic. Thus, nuclear enlargement and pleomorphism are seen along with clumping of the chromatin, increased nucleolar size and the appearance of double-nucleated cells [1, 2, 8, 10]. Cytoplasmic changes include irregularity and reduced numbers of acinar mitochondria plus loss of uniformity of the Golgi [21] and a reduced endoplasmic reticulum [8]. There is also an age-related increase in cells containing small or degenerating secretory granules [8, 18]. Intracytoplasmic vacuoles, increasing with age, have also been described [1, 18]. Since these vacuoles consist of lipid they are discussed more fully in the section on fatty changes below.

Histochemical studies on the rat submandibular gland have shown that the structural impairments are accompanied by age-related decreases in the amount of demonstrable enzymes in the acinar cells as well as in RNA and basic nucleoprotein [7]. On the other hand, despite the extent of these structural, enzymatic and biochemical defects, it has often proved difficult to demonstrate age differences in the quantity or composition of rat submandibular secretions. This suggests the presence in younger age groups of a substantial reserve capacity within the mass of secretory tissues of these glands.

Oncocytes

One of the features that has attracted most comment in accounts of aging in salivary glands is the occurrence of morphologically distinctive, probably inactive, cells referred to by Hamperl [16] as oncocytes. These cells are of swollen appearance, often with bulging outlines. They have strongly eosinophilic, slightly granular, cytoplasm with a central, vesicular or pyknotic nucleus (fig. 4). Occasionally binucleate forms occur.

Their ultrastructure is characterised by dense cytoplasmic accumulations of mitochondria and the loss of specialised cytoplasmic structures. Although initially the abundant closely packed mitochondria are all of normal morphology these organelles gradually assume a distorted appearance [8, 36].

Fig. 1. The contrasting general histology of young and old human submandibular glands. *a* Gland from a male aged 18 years showing an even, compact arrangement of the parenchyma with little adipose and fibrous tissues. *b* Gland from an 87-year-old male showing a less uniform and compact arrangement of the parenchyma with proportionally more adipose and fibrous tissue. Note in particular the prominence and dilatation of the ducts and their abundant fibrous surrounds. *A*, and *B*: both HE. Both × 28.

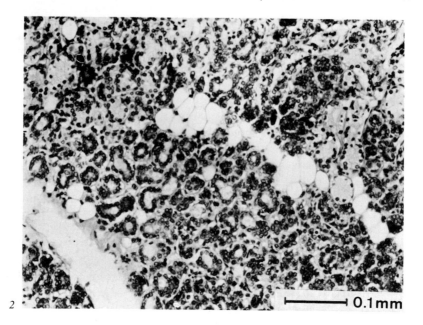

2   ⊢————⊣ 0.1mm

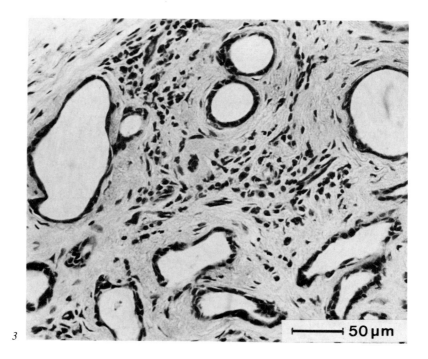

3   ⊢————⊣ 50 µm

Oncocytes occur singly or in clusters. Sometimes the latter consist of large hyperplastic foci and occasionally this change is sufficiently extensive as to replace an entire lobule. Oncocytic foci are also sometimes seen at the centres of lobules otherwise replaced by adipose tissue. At a histological level oncocytes appear to arise frequently from intercalated or striated ducts [4, 26, 31] but undoubtedly these cells also arise by transformations of acinar cells [16, 26]. Ultrastructural studies of human submandibular glands, in fact, have shown oncocytes arising most often from the acini and have confirmed the occurrence of transitional forms [36]. In the aging rat submandibular gland, on the other hand, the oncocytes appear to arise mainly from the intercalated ducts [8].

Oncocytes increase in frequency with increasing age both in the rat submandibular gland [8, 21] and in human major [3, 4, 16, 26] and minor glands [16, 31, 33, 34]. Although in man these cells are infrequently seen below 30 years they are almost invariably present after the age of 70 years [16, 26, 34]. However, oncocytes are not solely related to aging. They are a prominent feature of salivary tumours, most notably adenolymphoma and oxyphilic adenoma, the so-called oncocytoma, and they may also be associated with dilatation and cystic obstruction of the salivary ducts [35]. Moreover, oncocytes also occur in many exocrine and endocrine glands other than the salivary glands where also they are predominantly associated with aging.

The sporadic distribution of oncocytes alongside apparently functionally intact cells and their bizarre ultrastructural features attest to the non-functional character of oncocytes. They are, therefore, regarded as the end result of a specific type of degenerative change. The fact that once this degeneration has taken place, no further degenerative changes occur, together with their evident retention of the faculty of reproduction, explains the increasing prevalence of oncocytes with increasing age [16].

Age-Related Accumulations of Fat

Fat may accumulate in aging salivary glands by two independent mechanisms: as an increase of lipid droplets within the parenchymal cells or by an increase of mature adipose cells within the connective tissues of the glands.

Fig. 2. Atrophy and dedifferentiation of submandibular acini in a female aged 93 years. Degranulation and shrinkage of acinar cells has resulted in the appearance of numerous duct-like structures. HE. × 167.

Fig. 3. Part of a labial minor salivary gland lobule from a male aged 79 years; this field shows severe duct dilatation. No acini remain. They have been replaced by fibrous tissue with a mild patchy chronic inflammatory infiltrate. HE. × 280.

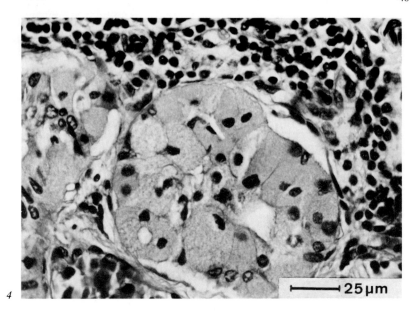

4   25 µm

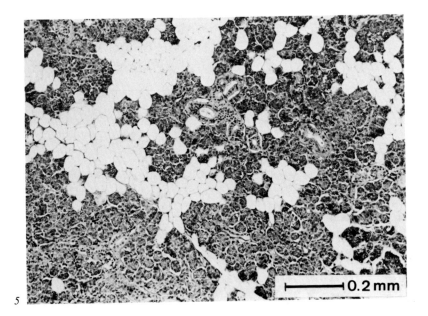

5   0.2 mm

Intracellular lipid droplets have been observed at the light microscope level in the acini and ducts of both human and rat major glands [1, 14, 38] where they appear to increase with age. They consist mainly of neutral fat and their presence has been confirmed by electron microscopy in man [15] and in the rat [8, 18]. Some of the lipid droplets are associated with the pigment lipofuscin. This material gradually accumulates with age in many tissues and organs, generally without any impairment of cellular function. In human salivary glands the lipofuscin is found in the striated ducts and gradually increases with age [15, 38]. In the rat parotid acinar cells lipofuscin granules increase with age until they occupy 2% of cell volume at 36 months of age [18].

In the major salivary glands of man fat accumulation occurs predominantly as progressive fatty infiltration which increases with age [3, 4, 14, 16, 26, 37]. In this process mature adipose cells accumulate in the septa and gradually encroach on the parenchyma extending inwards from the peripheries of the lobules (fig. 5). Sometimes entire lobules become replaced by adipose tissue in this way. This process occurs most excessively in the aging parotid gland but it may also be found in many submandibular glands in old age [14, 26]. It has recently also been reported in the serous glands of the tongue [11]. By contrast, it is less extensive in aging labial glands [12, 31]. The amount of adipose tissue, which is widely variable from gland to gland in any age group, has been shown to be independent of the general adiposity of the subject [37]. The reason for this adipose proliferation with age is unknown although it has been suggested that it may be linked to gradual losses by cell death in the parenchyma [14]. The earlier view that the adipose cells originate by fatty degeneration of parenchymal cells is now discounted [14].

Increased amounts of adipose tissue are also a feature of aging in the rat parotid [1, 19] but not in the rat submandibular or sublingual glands [2, 32]. However, assessment of the true extent of adipose accumulation in the rat parotid gland is difficult as the boundaries of this gland are poorly defined and the gland itself is enclosed by adipose tissue.

Fig. 4. Oncocytes in a submandibular intralobular duct in a male aged 91 years. Note the characteristic bulging granular cytoplasm and the variegated appearance of the nuclei. These cells may be found in the salivary glands of man at any age but they increase in frequency with age. HE. ×520. [From Ref. 24].

Fig. 5. Fatty infiltration of the submandibular gland in old age. Note the apparent origin of this process in the septa and the mature adipose cells extending centrally to replace or displace intralobular parenchymal elements. HE. × 79.

Age-Related Fibrosis

Throughout all salivary glands there is a fine network of supporting connective tissues extending from the capsule, where present, to interlobular septa and thence intralobularly to surround the individual parenchymal elements. Centrally the main collecting ducts are also ensheathed in fibrous tissue which again is continuous with the fine intralobular fibrillar network. In many types of salivary gland there is an age-related increase in the amount and density of this fibrous skeletal component both around the ducts and in the septa, which thus appear widened (fig. 1), and intralobularly so that the acini become slightly more widely spaced. These changes are particularly well developed in man especially in the aging submandibular gland [3, 14, 26] labial glands [12, 31] and the mucous glands of the tongue [11]. In the human parotid fibrosis also occurs with age but in most subjects it is overshadowed by the increasing adiposity. Fibrosis occurs with age in rat salivary glands [1, 32] but is limited in extent and hence more difficult to detect by subjective observation alone. It has not been found in aging rat sublingual glands [32].

As well as increasing in amount with age the connective tissue component of the salivary glands also exhibits altered histological characteristics. The collagen fibres become denser, more fragmented and less evenly orientated and elastic fibres are more numerous, thicker and fragmented. Prominent elastosis of the connective tissue sheaths of the extralobular ducts is an occasional finding in human submandibular glands after the age of 75 years and intralobular elastic tissue, rarely seen in young glands, is frequently encountered especially around striated ducts [26].

Lymphocytic Infiltration and Focal Lymphocytic Adenitis

Irrespective of age human and animal salivary glands contain lymphocytes, plasma cells, and histiocytes widely dispersed throughout the supporting tissues as a normal histological feature. In rat salivary glands mast cells are also a prominent feature. Periductal infiltrations of lymphocytes and plasma cells and the occurrence of proliferating foci of lymphocytic cells plus increased prevalence of mast cells have been reported as aging changes in the parotid and submandibular glands of the rat [1, 2].

Focal intralobular collections of lymphocytic cells, usually in a periductal location, are frequently present in human major salivary glands [3, 14, 16, 26, 37]. They are more prevalent in females, particularly over the age of 45 years [9] but generally do not show a consistent pattern of increasing prevalence over the full adult life span [24]. Likewise, focal or diffuse lymphocytic involvement of the minor glands [9, 20, 31] appears unrelated to aging although again more intense infiltration of the labial glands occurs in middle-aged females [9].

Focal Obstructive Adenitis

Small, usually well demarcated, areas of parenchymal degeneration with associated fibrosis and a variable degree of chronic inflammatory infiltration occur with increasing frequency in the major glands of man as age increases [16, 24]. Because the histological appearances often resemble those which occur throughout the gland after obstruction of a major duct, they have been referred to as focal obstructive adenitis in distinction from the focal lymphocytic adenitis of the previous section to which, it is stressed, they are unrelated [24]. The parenchymal changes in these lesions consist of acinar atrophy and/or dedifferentiation with loss of secretory granules, dilatation and hyperplasia of the ducts and a chronic inflammatory infiltration of variable intensity (fig. 6). In long-standing foci few remnants of the parenchyma can be found so that the area resembles a circumscribed fibrous scar often with few chronic inflammatory cells remaining [24]. The relationship of focal obstructive adenitis to age in human submandibular glands is shown in figure 7. In this series the mean number of foci per unit sectional area increased almost 8-fold over eight decades of human adult life.

Similar foci have been seen in human parotid glands in old age where they tend to include adipose tissue and in aging human labial glands [12, 31] where they may involve entire lobules. Also, similar focal changes occur in the submandibular glands of old rats but much less frequently than in human glands [32].

The focal changes, as described in the human submandibular gland (fig. 6), reflect in miniature the generalised response of the whole gland to aging, namely a degeneration and atrophy of parenchymal elements with replacement by connective tissues. The frequent occurrence of ductal dilatation in many such foci suggests that partial obstruction of the draining ducts may be responsible for the changes. Their increasing prevalence with age may reflect a reduced capacity for resolution by the damaged salivary epithelium in older age groups as well as an increasing incidence of obstruction to outflow, possibly by compression of the collecting ducts from the greater volume of fibro-adipose tissues present in the lobules of old glands.

Intraductal Deposits

In both the major and minor glands of man small plugs of apparently solid material are occasionally observed in the intralobular ducts. Although present in all age groups they are more common in old age [29, 31]. Similar consolidated material has been reported also in the parotid glands of old rats [1]. The number of deposits in the submandibular gland has been measured in human subjects of different ages [29]. The mean

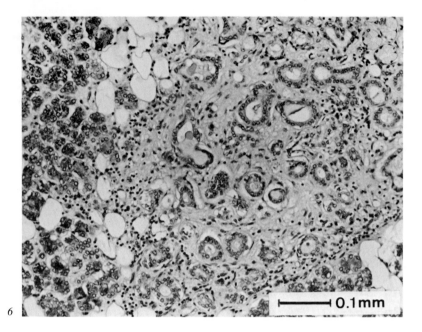

6

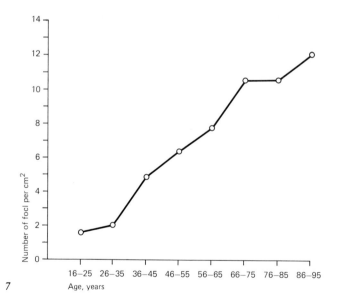

7

Table I. The mean prevalence of consolidated intraductal deposits in submandibular glands from subjects in four age groups

Age group years	Number of subjects	Number of deposits per cm^2 [a]	
		mean	SE
16–35	12	1.12	0.67
36–55	12	2.39	0.82
56–75	12	3.49	0.87
76–95	12	5.47	1.05

[a] Section areas were determined by point counting. The minimum area acceptable in the series was 1.5 cm^2.

prevalence increased almost 5-fold over the four 20-year age groups from 16 to 95 years (table I).

The deposits are of varied appearance. The majority are predominantly or entirely eosinophilic but some are haematoxyphilic and these may be calcified. Most of the deposits have a granular structureless appearance but some are concentrically laminated and appear to have formed about a central nidus (fig. 8). The deposits are mostly present in the lumens of the intralobular ducts but sometimes occur in the epithelial lining or even entirely in the connective tissues, as a result perhaps of atrophy of the original ductal epithelium. They also occur in the extra-lobular ducts and, rarely, in the acini. Sometimes these deposits are found in association with focal obstructive adenitis where they develop in the dilated ducts of the foci, probably as a consequence of stagnant flow in these areas [24, 29].

The deposits probably form by precipitation of salivary glycoprotein. This might be induced by alterations in electrolyte concentration in the ductal saliva, particularly in conditions of stagnation, or alternatively by mild disturbances of protein synthesis in the acinar cells. Both of these

Fig. 6. Focal obstructive adenitis in the submandibular gland from a 93-year-old male. This is a small focal area of intralobular fibrosis and ductal dilatation and hyperplasia. A few degenerate acini remain towards the lower part of the field and there is a mild chronic inflammatory infiltrate around the periphery of the focus. HE. × 139.

Fig. 7. The prevalence of focal obstructive adenitis in human submandibular glands in eight decades of adult age. The numbers of foci were counted in histological sections and the section areas were then derived from point counting. There were at least 5 males and 5 females in each age group. The mean index (number of foci per cm^2 per decade of age) shows a progressive increase over successive age decades. [From Ref. 24].

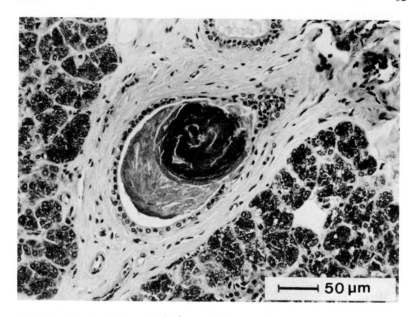

Fig. 8. An intraductal deposit of solid material in a small interlobular duct in a human submandibular gland. The deposit, which is concentrically laminated, appears to have formed around a central nidus. Such deposits occur at all ages but their prevalence increases with age. HE. × 213.

possibilities might be attributable to the structural changes which occur in parenchyma with increasing age. Although the histological structure of the laminated deposits appears similar to that of salivary calculi, the large number of microdeposits in older age groups is not accompanied by an increased incidence of sialolithiasis in old age. Clearly in all age groups, the great majority of microdeposits are easily voided in the saliva.

Quantitative Age Changes in Salivary Structure

Most of the quantitative studies on age changes in salivary structure have been carried out on human salivary glands obtained post mortem. Inevitably, therefore, the populations studied both within and between different series have been widely heterogeneous, particularly in respect of medical and therapeutic histories, causes of death, nutritional background, smoking and drinking habits, and dental status including the presence or absence of dentures. Although in most series so far reported attempts have been made to control for some of these variables, e.g. by using 'sudden death' cases and excluding particular drug medications and diseases, this has at best been only partially successful. Nevertheless, the strict application of excluding criteria employed in many of the investigations has probably avoided the seriously biased variability between age groups which characterised some of the earlier aging studies of salivary function and led to erroneous conclusions [5].

The quantitative methods employed have mostly utilised the stereological point-counting technique of assessing proportional volumes of salivary constituents, e.g. acini, ducts, adipose tissue. Interpretation of results has to be guarded, therefore, where proportional volumetric changes are unsupported by firm evidence for changes in the total gland volume. For example, the report of an apparent age-dependent decrease in a particular tissue may simply reflect an increase in other gland components in an enlarging gland. However, it is worth noting that for human salivary glands there is no evidence for an increase in size with age [12, 31, 37]. Indeed, where gland weight or volume has been measured, the evidence suggests a tendency for a reduced volume beyond the age of 75 years [23]. It is likely, therefore, that where systematic measurement has recorded relative losses in salivary parenchyma with increasing age, these studies do reflect an actual reduction in the true volume of tissue available for participation in secretory function.

Quantitative Age Changes in the Structure of Human Submandibular Glands

The submandibular is the only gland for which data are available for weight and volume over the human adult life span [23, 37]. As can be seen in figure 9 there is virtually no change in gland volume throughout most of adult life although the range at all ages is rather wide. However, beyond 75 years these data show a definite trend towards shrinkage of the glands as age rises further. In a statistical analysis of this data it was found that the volume reduction in the over-75-year age group was significant in females although not in males. Analysis of a series of 96 intact, non-diseased, formalin-fixed submandibular glands confirmed that for each of the sexes both the gland weight and volume were significantly reduced in the over-75-year age group but were unaffected by age differences in each of three 20-year age groups below 75 years [25].

Stereological analyses of healthy human submandibular glands have revealed that at around 20 years of age the parenchyma occupies approximately 70% of the gland volume. This then undergoes a steady decline with increasing age so that by about 90 years it occupies, on average, only some 50% of total gland volume [27, 37]. Since, as we have just seen,

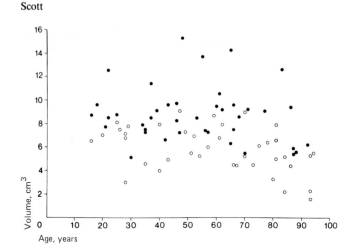

Fig. 9. Scatter diagram of submandibular gland volume in 39 males (●) and 41 females (○). The freshly dissected right gland was cleaned of excess connective tissue and the volume measured by a method of differential weighings in air and during immersion in a fluid of known specific gravity. There is a wide range of values for each sex at all ages but note the tendency for shrinkage over the last two decades.

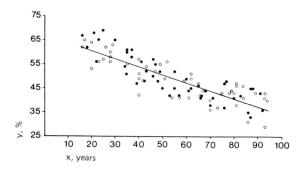

Fig. 10. Scatter diagram to show the age-related reduction in proportional volume of acinar tissue which occurs in human submandibular glands. The acinar volume (y) expressed as percentage of total gland volume was obtained by point counting and is plotted against age (x) in years for a total of 96 subjects, males (●) and females (○). The regression line, y = a + bx, has been fitted by calculation of the constants, a = 67.2 and b = −0.33, for which t = 15.6; p < 0.001.

Table II. Proportional volumes of component tissues (%) of human submandibular glands in decades of age

Decade years	Number	Acini mean (SE)	Ducts mean (SE)	Adipose mean (SE)	Other[a] mean (SE)
16–25	12	62.0 (1.50)	8.4 (0.37)	4.3 (0.99)	25.4 (1.03)
26–35	11	58.5 (1.26)	9.2 (0.43)	5.5 (1.74)	27.0 (1.35)
36–45	12	52.0 (1.57)	9.6 (0.34)	8.2 (1.65)	30.5 (1.02)
46–55	13	49.8 (1.44)	9.8 (0.42)	8.4 (1.99)	32.0 (2.04)
56–65	12	46.2 (1.10)	10.2 (0.49)	9.9 (1.51)	33.8 (0.98)
66–75	11	40.7 (0.80)	10.7 (0.60)	10.4 (2.08)	38.2 (2.08)
76–85	13	43.4 (0.97)	11.3 (0.53)	13.0 (2.45)	32.3 (1.81)
86–95	12	38.5 (1.59)	10.6 (0.55)	15.1 (1.47)	35.8 (2.38)

[a] Predominantly fibrous and vascular tissues.

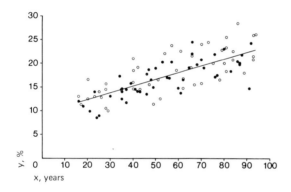

Fig. 11. Scatter diagram to show the age-related increase in ductal volume relative to total parenchyma in human submandibular glands. Acinar (A) and ductal (D) proportional volumes were obtained by point counting. The value of y is $\dfrac{D}{A + D}$ expressed as percentage and that of x is age in years. For the regression line, y = a + bx, a = 9.46 and b = 0.14 for which t = 11.1; p < 0.001. There were 96 subjects, males (●) and females (○).

there is no enlargement of the gland through adult life these findings reflect a true loss of glandular epithelium with age. Moreover, it has also been shown that this loss occurs entirely within the acinar component (fig. 10) because concomitantly there is a progressive rise in the proportional volume of ducts with age (table II). These progressive but opposite

Table III. Proportion of total duct volume (%) occupied by different categories of ducts in human submandibular glands in decades of age

Decade years	Number	Extralobular mean (SE)	Intralobular (striated) mean (SE)	Intralobular (non-striated) mean (SE)
16–25	9	10.1 (0.94)	60.2 (2.33)	29.7 (1.57)
26–35	9	11.8 (0.92)	59.2 (1.82)	29.0 (2.08)
36–45	10	11.8 (1.03)	58.1 (2.09)	30.0 (2.50)
46–55	10	13.6 (1.30)	51.8 (1.74)	34.6 (1.84)
56–65	11	11.2 (0.66)	51.1 (2.06)	37.7 (2.03)
66–75	9	15.8 (2.56)	44.6 (2.37)	39.7 (1.80)
76–85	12	16.2 (1.98)	44.8 (2.69)	39.0 (2.61)
86–95	12	18.3 (1.39)	40.7 (2.18)	41.0 (1.55)

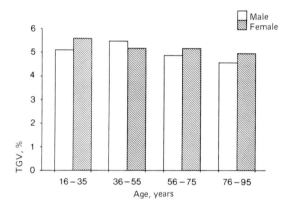

Fig. 12. Histogram to show the mean proportion of total submandibular gland volume (TGV) occupied by striated ducts in four successive 20-year age groups. The volume proportions were obtained by point counting. At least 10 males and 10 females were included in each age group. Unlike other gland components, the striated ducts maintain a constant proportion of gland volume across the four age groups. The small differences in column heights were not statistically significant.

changes account for the prominence of ducts frequently observed in older glands. The contrasting relationship of acini and ducts to aging is further depicted in figure 11. In this series the ratio of ducts to total parenchyma increased almost 2-fold between 20 and 90 years. However, ducts account for only a small fraction of the complete gland and the severe loss of the main component, the acini, is compensated for largely by changes in the fibro-vascular and adipose components (table II).

The age-related increase in the proportional volume of the ducts does not take place evenly in all categories of ducts. In the human submandibular glands a close analysis of volumetric changes in the ducts alone [28] showed that most of the increase could be accounted for by changes in the volume proportion of non-striated intralobular ducts (table III), corresponding therefore with the hyperplasia, metaplasia, oncocytosis and dilatation already noted in the descriptive accounts above. An increase in proportional volume also occurred in the extralobular ducts although this was mostly restricted to the age groups above 65 years. An important finding emerging from this study was that for the striated ducts the proportional volume remained almost constant at about 5% of gland volume over all age groups (fig. 12). In old age, therefore, not only is there a greater total volume of ducts, but relative to the acinar volume, there is also a higher volume of striated ducts. This is available for processing the output of a diminished quantity of acinar tissue and may be important, therefore, in ensuring the maintenance of a hypotonic saliva in old age when the structural derangements of the other intralobular elements might otherwise impair this faculty.

In general, the stereological analyses of the human submandibular gland confirm the earlier subjective accounts of acinar loss, ductal proliferation, fibrosis and adiposity of the glands in old age. They also show quite clearly that these changes are gradual and progressive throughout the whole of adult life. Together with the results of a complementary study of the submandibular glands in childhood and adolescence, in which no deteriorative features were revealed [30], they point to the onset of aging deterioration occurring in early adulthood soon after the development and growth of the gland is completed. The progressive reduction in the actual volume of acinar tissue in the submandibular gland, amounting to over one third of that initially present in the young adult, provides us with a rational explanation for the reduced salivary flow which is the chief functional characteristic of these glands in old age [22; Baum, this volume].

Quantitative Age Changes in the Structure of Human Parotid Glands
The parotid gland is the largest of the human salivary glands and its deep lobe is also the most inaccessible. For this reason there is little quantitative data available to indicate the nature and extent of any structural responses to aging in the parotid. In a preliminary study in the author's laboratory, using the superficial lobe of the parotid from 30 subjects at necropsy, aged 17–90 years, the mean proportional volumes of parenchymal and adipose tissues were determined by a stereological analysis. This was restricted to the intralobular tissues. The outstanding feature of

Table IV. Proportional volumes of intralobular component tissues (%) of human parotid glands in three age groups

Age group years	Number	Parenchyma[a] mean (SE)	Adipose mean (SE)	Other[b] mean (SE)
17–40	8	65.8 (3.09)	24.5 (2.94)	9.7 (0.71)
41–69	10	64.8 (4.84)	24.8 (5.42)	10.4 (1.17)
70–90	12	53.3 (4.02)	36.8 (4.83)	9.8 (1.17)

[a] Acini and ducts.
[b] Predominantly fibrous and vascular tissue.

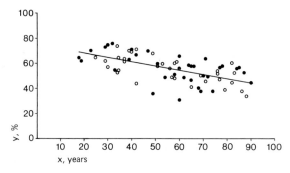

Fig. 13. Scatter diagram to illustrate the age-related reduction of parenchymal tissue which occurs in human labial glands. The proportional volume of parenchyma (y) was obtained by point counting and is expressed as a percentage of the labial gland volume. Males (●) and females (○) are depicted separately in the total of 68 subjects. The slope of the regression line, y = a + bx, is highly significant: a = 74.23, b = –0.325, for which t = 5.8; $p < 0.001$.

this small series was the high level of adiposity encountered at all age groups. The results are given in table IV. It can be seen that the proportional volume of parenchyma was significantly reduced by 20% of its own initial value between the youngest and oldest age groups (t = 2.25). This was almost entirely compensated for by an increase in the mean proportional volume of adipose tissue. However, the variance in all groups was extremely wide and with the small numbers available the increase in adipose content approached, but failed to achieve, significance at the 5% level (t = 1.93). In the absence of direct evidence about changes in total gland volume with age it is not possible to infer true losses of acinar tissue from these proportional volumetric changes, even though degenerative acinar changes of dedifferentiation and atrophy, resembling

Table V. Proportional volumes of component tissues (%) of human labial salivary glands in three age groups

Age group years	Number	Acini mean (SE)	Ducts mean (SE)	Other tissue[a] mean (SE)
18–40	20	56.6 (1.93)	8.5 (0.92)	34.9 (1.59)
41–65	24	40.8 (2.81)	14.1 (1.58)	45.2 (2.15)
66–90	24	32.1 (2.40)	17.4 (1.10)	50.5 (1.71)

[a] Other tissues consist mainly of fibrous and vascular tissues and include adipose tissue. This was less than 5% in most glands.

those in the submandibular gland, were seen in the old parotids. It is of interest, therefore, that in recent closely controlled investigations of parotid flow, no aging differences were demonstrable in either stimulated or resting secretions [6, 17]. If some actual loss of acinar volume does, in fact, take place with age it would seem to be too small to influence parotid function at a clinically detectable level.

Quantitative Age Changes in the Structure of Human Minor Salivary Glands

The most accessible group of minor salivary glands in man are those located superficially between the mucosa and the muscle in the lower lip. These glands have been widely studied in disease and recently their structure has been analysed in relation to aging [12, 31]. In a series of 68 subjects aged 18–90 years examined at necropsy, after excluding drug medications or diseases likely to influence salivary structure, it was found that the proportional volume of labial salivary parenchyma underwent a progressive decline with increasing age (fig. 13). As in the submandibular glands, this change occurred within the acinar component (table V) while the ductal proportional volume doubled between the young and old age groups. The lost acinar tissue was replaced mainly by fibro-vascular tissues while adipose infiltration was only rarely seen [31]. These findings have been closely confirmed by other quantitative studies of labial glands [12] and, furthermore, the same author has recently reported similar quantitative differences in aging human lingual glands [11].

In the series described here the number of transected salivary gland lobules in standard-sized midline lower labial specimens varied widely across the age range but did not differ significantly between the three age groups defined in table V. Thus, in the absence of any evidence suggesting an increase in the total number of labial salivary lobules with age, it is likely that the age-dependent reduction in proportional acinar volume represents a true loss of secretory acinar tissue. This loss which amounts to more than 40% of the acinar tissue present in the young age group provides a structural explanation for the recent report of an age-related decrease in labial salivary flow rate [13].

Aging and Age-Related Pathology in Salivary Glands

Aging in the salivary glands, as elsewhere, comprises a complex series of inter-related processes which progressively lead towards a breakdown of tissue integrity and a loss of functional capacity. Moreover, these processes overlap and inter-react with instances of age-related disease within the glands.

In human salivary glands the presence of degenerative vascular disease is an almost constant finding in middle-aged and older subjects [26]. The extent to which this results in a progressive impairment of the capillary blood supply to individual parenchymal units has not been investigated, but it is reasonable to assume that it gives rise to some degree of ischaemia within the glands. This, therefore, suggests a rational explanation for the age-dependent deterioration of the glands, whereby highly specialised and metabolically active secretory epithelium involutes and is replaced by more inert fibro-adipose tissue in which the requirement for high levels of blood supply are much reduced. It would be mistaken, however, to regard the extensive losses of salivary parenchyma in old age as being entirely the result of atherosclerosis and related vascular diseases. Parenchymal aging losses may also occur in occasional human glands where deterioration of the vessels is minimal and are present, for instance, in the rat [32] where vascular disease in old age is generally insignificant.

Other more minor pathological changes are also seen with increasing frequency in older salivary glands. The foci of obstructive adenitis and the intraductal deposits already described are examples. So too is the ductal dilatation noted in the labial glands. While these small areas of actual or potential tissue damage are outside the range of normal biological variation, as we have seen they are, nonetheless, almost universally present in older glands. They illustrate the close relation between pathological events and the progressive structural degradation of aging. Thus, inherent aging in the epithelium may render glandular elements more vulnerable to environmental stress, such as that occasioned by gradual impairment of the blood supply. Concomitantly, specialised epithelium damaged by trauma or infection retains a reduced ability for healing through regeneration. In each case the combined result is progressive loss of glandular epithelium.

The two phenomena, aging and age-associated disease, therefore, are quantitative variables of salivary structure which influence each other and may be synergistic in their effects. In this sense salivary structural aging can be regarded as a state of ongoing low-grade pathological change. Failure in its containment ultimately leads to a loss of function, while the passage of time increases the likelihood that such failure will occur.

References

1   Andrew, W.: Age changes in the parotid glands of Wistar Institute rats with special reference to the occurrence of oncocytes in senility. Am. J. Anat. *85:* 157–197 (1949).

2   Andrew, W.: Age changes in the salivary glands of Wistar Institute rats with particular reference to the submandibular glands. J. Geront. *4:* 95–103 (1949).

3   Andrew, W.: A comparison of age changes in salivary glands of man and of the rat. J. Geront. *7:* 178–190 (1952).

4   Bauer, W. H.: Old age changes in human parotid glands with special reference to peculiar cells in uncommon salivary gland tumors (Abstract). J. dent. Res. *29:* 686 (1950).

5   Baum, B. J.: Research on aging and oral health: an assessment of current status and future needs. Spec. Care Dent. *1:* 156–165 (1981).

6   Baum, B. J.: Evaluation of stimulated parotid saliva flow rate in different age groups. J. dent. Res. *60:* 1292–1296 (1981).

7   Bogart, B. I.: The effect of aging on the histochemistry of the rat submandibular gland. J. Geront. *22:* 372–375 (1967).

8   Bogart, B. I.: The effect of aging in the rat submandibular gland: an ultrastructural, cytochemical and biochemical study. J. Morph. *130:* 337–352 (1970).

9   Chisholm, D. M.; Waterhouse, J. P.; Mason, D. K.: Lymphocytic sialadenitis in the major and minor glands: a correlation in postmortem subjects. J. clin. Path. *23:* 690–694 (1970).

10 Church, E. L.: Age changes in the nucleus of salivary glands of Wistar Institute rats. Oral Surg. *8:* 301–314 (1955).

11 Drummond, J. R.: A histological study of structural changes occurring in the human lingual minor salivary glands in old age (Abstract). J. dent. Res. *64:* 681 (1985).

12 Drummond, J. R.; Chisholm, D. M.: A qualitative and quantitative study of the ageing human labial salivary glands. Archs oral Biol. *29:* 151–155 (1984).

13 Gandara, B. K.; Izutsu, K. T.; Truelove, E. L.; Ensign, W. Y.; Sommers, E. E.: Age-related salivary flow rate changes in controls and patients with oral lichen planus. J. dent. Res. *64:* 1149–1151 (1985).

14 Garrett, J. R.: Some observations on human submandibular salivary glands. Proc. R. Soc. Med. *55:* 488–491 (1962).

15 Garrett, J. R.: The ultrastructure of intracellular fat in the parenchyma of human sub-mandibular salivary glands. Archs oral Biol. *8:* 729–734 (1963).

16 Hamperl, H.: Beiträge zur normalen und pathologischen Histologie menschlicher Speicheldrüsen. Z. Zellforsch. *27:* 1–55 (1931).

17 Heft, M. W.; Baum, B. J.: Unstimulated and stimulated parotid salivary flow rate in individuals of different ages. J. dent. Res. *63:* 1182–1185 (1984).

18   Kim, S. K.: Changes in the secretory acinar cells of the rat parotid gland during aging. Anat. Rec. *209:* 345–354 (1984).

19   Kim, S. K.; Weinhold, P. A.; Han, S. S.; Wagner, D. J.: Age-related decline in protein synthesis in the rat parotid gland. Exp. Gerontol. *15:* 77–85 (1980).

20   Kingsbury, B. F.: Lymphatic tissue and regressive structure with particular reference to degeneration of glands. Am. J. Anat. *77:* 159–187 (1945).

21   Kurtz, S. M.: Cytologic studies of the salivary glands of the rat in reference to the aging process. J. Geront. *9:* 421–428 (1954).

22   Pedersen, W.; Schubert, M.; Izutsu, K.; Mersai, T.: Truelove, E.: Age-dependent decreases in human submandibular gland flow rates as measured under resting and post-stimulation conditions. J. dent. Res. *64:* 822–825 (1985).

23   Scott, J.: Age, sex and contralateral differences in the volumes of human submandibular salivary glands. Archs oral Biol. *20:* 885–887 (1975).

24   Scott, J.: The incidence of focal chronic inflammatory changes in human submandibular salivary glands. J. oral Pathol. *5:* 334–346 (1976).

25   Scott, J.: Aging in the human submandibular gland: a morphometric study; PhD thesis, Liverpool (1976).

26   Scott, J.: Degenerative changes in the histology of the human submandibular salivary gland occurring with age. J. Biol. buccale *5:* 311–319 (1977).

27   Scott, J.: Quantitative age changes in the histological structure of human submandibular salivary glands. Archs oral Biol. *22:* 221–227 (1977).

28   Scott, J.: A morphometric study of age changes in the histology of the ducts of human submandibular salivary glands. Archs oral Biol. *22:* 243–249 (1977).

29   Scott, J.: The prevalence of consolidated salivary deposits in the small ducts of human submandibular glands. J. oral Pathol. *7:* 28–37 (1978).

30   Scott, J.: Qualitative and quantitative changes in the histology of the human submandibular salivary gland during post natal growth. J. Biol. buccale *7:* 341–352 (1979).

31   Scott, J.: Qualitative and quantitative observations on the histology of human labial salivary glands obtained post mortem. J. Biol. buccale *8:* 187–200 (1980).

32   Scott, J.; Bodner, L.; Baum, B. J.: Assessment of age-related changes in the submandibular and sublingual salivary glands of the rat using stereological analysis. Archs oral Biol. *31:* 69–71 (1986).

33   Shimono, M.; Yamamura, T.: Ultrastructure of the oncocyte in normal human palatine salivary glands. J. Electron Microsc. *24:* 119–121 (1975).

34   Soames, J. V.: A review of the histology of the tongue in the region of the foramen caecum. Oral Surg. *36:* 220–224 (1973).

35   Southam, J. C.: Retention mucoceles of the oral mucosa. J. oral Pathol. *3:* 197–202 (1974).

36   Tandler, B.: Fine structure of oncocytes in human salivary glands. Virchows Arch. Abt. A Path. Anat. *341:* 317–326 (1966).

37   Waterhouse, J. P.; Chisholm, D. M.; Winter, R. B.; Patel, M.; Yale, R. S.: Replacement of functional parenchymal cells by fat and connective tissue in human submandibular salivary glands: an age-related change. J. oral Pathol. *2:* 16–27 (1973).

38   Yamaguchi, S.: Studien über die Mundspeicheldrüsen. 1. Über das Fett. Beitr. path. Anat. allg. Pathol. *73:* 113–122 (1925).

John Scott, BDS, PhD, School of Dental Surgery, The University of Liverpool, Liverpool L693BX (England)

Front. oral Physiol., vol. 6, pp. 63–84 (Karger, Basel 1987)

Changes in Innervation of Dentine and Pulp with Age

K. Fried

Department of Anatomy, Karolinska Institutet, Stockholm, Sweden

Introduction

In all mammalian species, including man, the dentition is continuously subject to wear and injury, perhaps to a larger extent than any other part of the body. As a result, various dental defects become more and more evident with increasing age [51]. It is obvious that such changes must affect the pulpal and dentinal innervation of the older tooth. Apart from this, changes may also occur in dental nerves due to other factors, e.g. mere biological aging. The important functional roles of the pulpal innervation, as a nociceptive system aimed at preserving the dentition, and/or as a mechanoreceptive device involved in mastication [19], motivates a detailed description of changes in tooth pulp axon morphology with age. This chapter summarizes such changes. In addition, several possible functional consequences of these structural changes are discussed. The description is based on light and electron microscopic studies in the cat performed in our laboratory [23]. These results, however, appear to have relevance to other mammalian systems as well, including man [cf. 39].

The fact that the subject is maturing or aging does not necessarily mean that it is in a unique state of development or that it is undergoing senescent deterioration [cf. 84]. In the young mammal, for example, the primary dentition, including its terminal innervation, undergoes a process which closely resembles a senescent transformation [28]. In the dentition of the aged mammals, on the other hand, various attempts at regeneration may be initiated by wear and injury [51]. For this reason, an account of dental innervation with aging would be incomplete without a brief description of pulpal axons present earlier in life. For a detailed information on early development, the reader is referred to other review articles [14, 22, 23, 38].

Development of Primary Tooth Pulp Axons

The primary tooth buds develop prenatally, but their dental papillae are in general very sparsely innervated [13, 61, 74], or not at all [28], until crown and root formation is well under way. Available evidence suggests that the primary tooth buds at a very early stage are surrounded by a plexus of axons from which, much later, terminal arbors enter the dental pulp [22, 28, 60, 61]. The mechanisms governing axon ingrowth into the tooth pulps are not well understood and need to be studied further.

The pioneer axons that enter the pulpal tissue shortly before tooth eruption are closely associated with pulpal blood vessels [22, 28]. Concomitant with eruption of the tooth, pulpal axons rapidly increase in number and myelination is initiated. When the formation and eruption of the primary dentition is completed and the root apices close, the pulpal innervation is fully developed [28].

Pulpal Axon Degeneration in Exfoliating Primary Teeth

Shortly after the pulpal axons have attained full maturity, the first signs of unmyelinated axon degeneration are found [28]. These include the appearance of swollen axons with an electron-lucent axoplasm that lacks most organelles. Some unmyelinated axons are apparently lost at this early stage. As root resorption advances an increasing proportion of unmyelinated axons are involved, and some myelinated axons also become affected. These display a loss of organelles, while the Schwann cell-myelin unit appears intact. Sometimes the axon disappears entirely, leaving a collapsed Schwann cell-myelin unit. In advanced stages, the Schwann cells degenerate as well and severely altered pulps may become completely denervated (fig. 1). This pattern of primary pulpal axon and Schwann cell degeneration is probably caused by local factors associated with tooth resorption. Biochemical changes produced by dentinoclast and fibroblast activities [2], as well as vascular changes which appear late during resorption [46], might be involved.

It is important to note that the inferior alveolar nerve (IAN), the stem nerve trunk supplying the mandibular dentition with pulpal axons, is structurally unaffected during the period of degeneration of the primary pulpal axons and the subsequent ingrowth of nerve fibres into the permanent teeth [23]. This indicates that the set of preterminal and terminal pulpal axon branches is very plastic and responsive to the remodelling of the dentition.

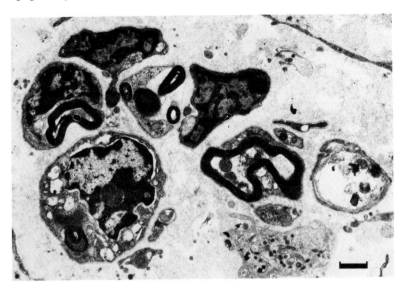

Fig. 1. Electron micrograph showing severely altered Schwann cell profiles, containing remnants of myelinated or unmyelinated axons, in highly resorbed feline primary incisor. Scale bar 1 μm. From ref. [28].

Development of Permanent Pulpal Axons

Prior to the time when signs of primary pulpal axon degeneration begin to become evident, the first axons have already begun to enter the permanent tooth pulp [29]. Simultaneously, the as-yet-unerupted permanent tooth develops a mineralized crown and root formation commences.

As in primary teeth, the developing permanent tooth bud appears to be closely associated with nerve fibre plexa without receiving any pulpal axons until later stages. The possibility that dental pulps attract axons through some trophic factor, released at a certain stage of tooth development, cannot be excluded. This proposed mechanism is supported by the observation that denervated dental pulps, in animals where the original nerve trunk is prevented from regenerating, become reinnervated by other adjacent nerves [67]. Additional evidence is provided by the fact that feline permanent incisor tooth buds, after being autotransplanted to hindlimbs, receive pulpal innervation from spinal nerves [20].

Continued permanent pulpal axon ingrowth, myelination and maturation proceeds pari passu with eruption, mineralization and root formation. The number of pulpal axons is established when the apical foramen of the tooth closes. The nerve bundles, which lack perineural sheaths, pass through the radicular pulp with little branching [14, 26] and then fan out in the coronal pulp and proceed to the pulp-dentine border [36]. At this stage of apical closure the plexus of Raschkow is formed and the terminals in the odontoblast layer, predentine and dentine are established. This process is initiated at the tip of the pulpal horn and spreads apically to other crown areas [13]. The morphological observation that axonal ingrowth into the pulp begins before and continues after eruption agrees with electrophysiological findings in the rat. Rat molar teeth show an increase in sensitivity during the eruptive period, measured using the digastric reflex response to electrical stimulation [14]. It is also in line with clinical observations: partly erupted teeth appear to be less sensitive to stimulation with an electric pulp tester than mature ones [33, 39, 44]. Morphological and functional studies thus confirm that sensory axon maturation in both apical and coronal-dentinal regions roughly coincides with closure of the apical foramen. Although permanent teeth usually contain a larger number of nerve fibres [29, 40; see, however, 38] the pattern of innervation in primary and permanent teeth is qualitatively similar. As in primary teeth, permanent pulpal axons are not initially surrounded by a perineurium [29, 56]. Quantitative parameters of myelinated and unmyelinated pulpal axons (other than total numbers) are also comparable, although myelinated axons in young adult permanent pulps may reach slightly larger sizes than in primary pulps.

Changes in Tooth Structure Related to Aging

Aging is accompanied by profound structural and chemical changes in the tooth [51, 53]. It is inevitable that some of these changes will affect pulpal innervation. In fact, there are reasons to believe that most of senescent pulpal axon pathology is invoked by environmental factors. Some of the changes in periodontal, calcified and pulpal tissues of the tooth that occur with aging are therefore summarized below. For a detailed description of these features the reader is referred to thorough reviews on the subject [8, 42, 51, 53].

Periodontal Tissue. Periodontal tissue recedes in the apical direction as age advances. This process is associated with changes in adjacent tissues, such as detachment and loosening of root surface fibres from the periodontal membrane, bony tooth socket resorption and atrophy of the gingival margin tissue [42, 51]. These alterations eventually result in various degrees of increased tooth motility. Although present in most older people, it is not clear whether these periodontal processes should be considered purely age-related or, alternatively, whether they are more closely related to the severity of the local inflammatory process.

Enamel. Apart from substance loss due to wear, the main change with age in enamel seems to be a slight alteration in the chemical composition of the outer layer [51]. According to some workers [45] the organic substance between the prisms becomes calcified in aging enamel. This may be the reason why enamel becomes more brittle and fractures more easily with increasing age [42].

Cementum. With increasing age there is a significant increase in thickness of cementum on the root [4]. This process divides and narrows the apical canals which convey the neurovascular bundles into the pulp [51]. Some older teeth also show signs of root resorption. This feature has been claimed to be positively correlated to increasing age, but it is probably, rather, a direct result of local injuries and mechanical stress.

Dentine. Primary dentine is subject to an age-related increasing mineralization that results in dentine sclerosis [4, 42, 51]. This is partly due to an attrition-related increase in peritubular dentine, eventually closing the lumen of many dentinal tubules [50]. The major age change in dentine is however the formation of regular or irregular secondary dentine due to physiological and pathological stimuli [51]. This process results in a gradual reduction in the size of the pulp chamber and root canals [e.g. 53]. The number of dentinal tubules is also reduced by this process since irregular secondary dentine, which is mainly deposited in the coronal regions, obliterates many tubule openings [42].

Dental Pulp. The dental pulp shows a reduction in number of fibroblasts and odontoblasts with age, as noted previously by Tomes [78; see also 9, 62] The odontoblast layer may also show intra- and intercellular vacuolization [48]. The number of vascular structures in the pulp decreases, mainly because of a reduction in sub-odontoblastic layer vessels [5]. There is an increase in the density of the fibrous component, probably a result of the persistence of fibrous elements in an originally larger pulp [9]. The incidence of pulpal calcification, either diffuse or in the form of nodules, increases with age [51, 62]. In some aging pulps a pronounced degradation of the tissue is evident; there are very few pulpal cells and vessels, the odontoblast layer is absent and most of the pulpal space is occupied by collagen and a flocculent material [29, 42].

Senescent Changes in the Innervation of Permanent Teeth

Subsequent to final maturation, which roughly coincides with closure of the apical foramen, the permanent pulpal axons enter a short, relatively stable stage [29]. During this period, the pulpal axons do not change significantly, apart from a slightly expanded myelinated axon size range and somewhat increased myelin sheath thicknesses. However, concomitant with the continued narrowing of the root canal and pulp chamber, a phase of axonal degeneration and loss inevitably follows. A light microscopically detectable loss of nerve fibres in aging constricted pulps was originally noted in human teeth by Tomes [78], and was subsequently confirmed in later studies: human [11] and rat [6]. Only more recently, however, has more detailed information on the structural alterations that pulpal axons undergo in old age emerged [23, 27]. When describing these events it appears appropriate to deal with the crown segment and the root canal segment of the pulpal axons separately. There are reasons to expect that many of the senescent axonal changes are related to environmental factors, e.g. attrition and changes in dental structure and function. The crown region is probably often affected first [13] and morphological abnormalities in the root region may to some extent be secondary to pulpal chamber injuries.

Crown Region. The pattern of axon trajectories through the dental pulp does not differ between young and old teeth. Intradental arborization commences at the crown pulp level in old age, although an actual pulpal widening may be hard to detect due to secondary dentine deposition [27]. The myelinated axons in the crown pulp core of aging teeth usually appear slightly atrophic and occasional Schwann cell protrusions into the axoplasm are found (see below). The total number of axons appears to be lower than at earlier stages since the size of the crown pulp has been reduced. However, clear-cut myelinated or unmyelinated axonal abnormalities are otherwise lacking [21, 37] (fig. 2). At the pulp-dentine border, it seems that the innervation of coronal dentine is modified by the increased rate of secondary dentine deposition. This modification includes a continued terminal branching of axons and enclosure of nerves within newly formed dentine [13, 37]. There is also a gradual loss of nerves at the tip of the cusp because of the formation of non-innervated reparative dentine [6, 13]. These events seem to cooperate in a process in which there is a gradual apical shift in the location of innervated dentine: from the tip of the cusp at eruption to mid-coronal dentine at midlife and dentine in the lower crown region of the aging tooth [13].

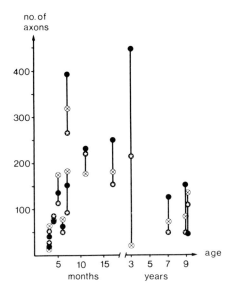

Fig. 2. Graph showing total number of axons in the apical root region of intact individual feline permanent incisors during development and aging (star = 1st incisor; x = 2nd incisor; filled circle = 3rd incisor). From ref. [29].

Apical Region. As the pulpal space constricts with age the number of pulpal axons usually decreases [9, 29, 39] (fig. 2). The size range of myelinated axons is similar to that in the young adult (fig. 3), but the myelin sheaths tend to be thicker (fig. 4).

Estimates of the proportion of myelinated to unmyelinated axons do not indicate any preferential loss of either of these axon types [29]. Qualitative electron microscopic observations (fig. 5a) show that signs of unmyelinated axon degeneration can be sometimes detected; degenerating myelinated fibres are rarely encountered. The degenerating unmyelinated axons appear swollen and lack neurotubuli, microfilaments and mitochondria. Collagen Schwann cell pockets occur, both in cells related to unmyelinated axons and in Schwann cells which lack an axonal relation (fig. 5c). The average number of unmyelinated axons per Schwann cell profile is a little lower than in young mature cats, and fewer larger unmyelinated axons are found [29, 39]. It is not known if the reaction of the population of sympathetic unmyelinated axons to aging is different from that of sensory axons. This does not seem likely, however. Myelinated axons appear smaller in relation to myelin sheath thickness than at earlier stages, giving the impression of axonal atrophy (fig. 5b). Schwann cell

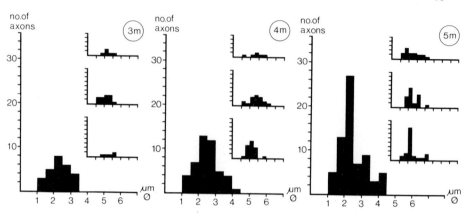

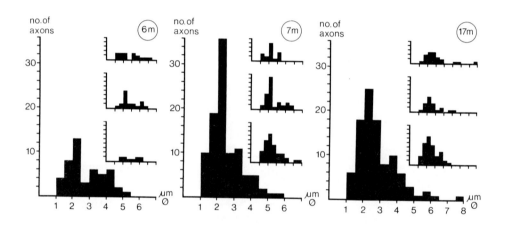

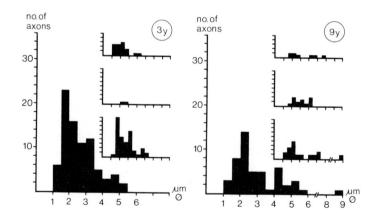

3

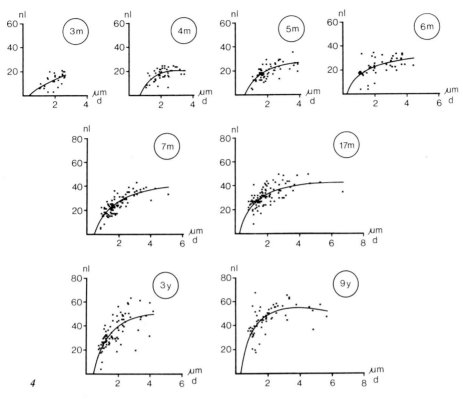

Fig. 4. Graphs showing the number of myelin lamellae (nl) plotted against axon diameter (d) of pulpal axons in the apical root region of feline permanent incisors at some developmental stages. In each case the line drawn illustrates the linear + logarithmic function which was found to be best adapted to observed values (m = months; y = years). From ref. [29].

Fig. 3. Size distribution of myelinated axons (including myelin sheaths) in the apical root region of intact feline permanent incisor pulps during development and aging. Large histograms represent pooled data from three ipsilateral intact incisors. Small histograms indicate size range in individual pulps (top = 1st incisor; middle = 2nd incisor; bottom = 3rd incisor) The scales in the small histograms correspond to those in the large ones (m = months; y = years). From ref. [29].

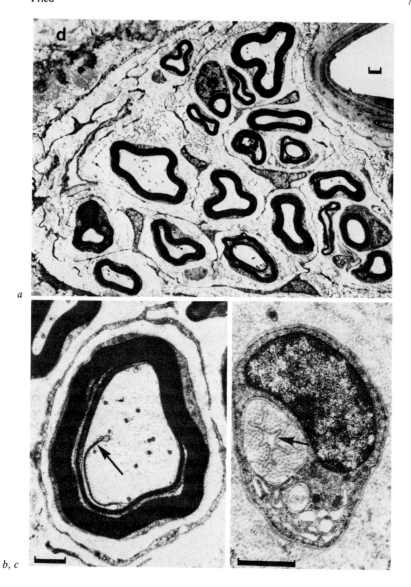

Fig. 5. Electron micrographs from transverse sections through the apical root region of aging (9 years) feline mandibular incisors. From ref. [29]. All scale bars 1 μm. *a* Survey micrograph of axons in a moderately narrowed pulp. *b* A myelinated axon, which is surrounded by a perineuriumlike sheath, is seen with a Schwann cell tongue extruding into the axoplasm (arrow). *c* This picture shows what seems to be a Schwann cell lacking an axonal relation. Note the basement membrane-covered pocket, which contains collagen and an additional, wrinkled basement membrane (arrow).

tongues can be seen extruding into the axoplasm, and some of these seem to develop into adaxonal networks encircling portions of axoplasm. Demyelinated axons are occasionally found, as well as very thinly myelinated fibres which seem to be remyelinating.

In teased fibre preparation of aging tooth pulps, myelinated fibres can be visualized over long intrapulpal distances [26, 27]. Such preparations usually yield a few exceptionally large fibres, with diameters up to 9 μm. These large axons often have nodes of Ranvier partly covered with myelin folds (fig. 7a) [cf. 57]. In general, however, very few axons with diameters above 4 μm are found in the aging pulp. Since nerve fibre diameter ranges up to ~ 7 μm in the young adult, aging must involve a selective loss of larger myelinated pulpal fibres and/or axonal atrophy. Also internodal lengths tend to be lower in the old pulp (fig. 6). This is probably a result of de- and remyelinating events [cf. 47, 58]. Qualitative signs of such myelin sheath remodelling are common. In addition to the characteristics of the larger axons which were mentioned above, many very short (10–50 μm) intercalated internodal segments occur on smaller sized axons. These consist mainly of three types: (1) smooth internodes with the Schwann cell nucleus in the middle of the segment, (2) smooth internodes with eccentric Schwann cell nuclei, and (3) distorted internodes with multiple myelin protrusions and swellings (fig. 7). In addition to intercalated internodes, many axons display myelin wrinkling, nodal lengthening and formation of myelin ovoids (fig. 7). Some axonal segments lack myelin in what appear to be former paranodal regions, suggesting demyelination [17, 18]. Signs of Wallerian degeneration are not usually present.

Nerve fibre changes similar to those described here have been encountered in peripheral nerves during aging in both experimental animals and humans [35, 47, 69, 71]. A number of possible causes have been suggested: biological aging as such, metabolic/toxic disease, dying-back processes, neuronal loss or distal nerve pressure lesions [see 35 for references]. Since similar changes can be elicited through nerve compression and also occur proximal to neurotomies and neuromas [1, 17, 54, 57, 73] degenerative nerve fibre changes have often been ascribed to age-related alterations of the target tissue, e.g. after prolonged pressure and irritation [35, 71, 76; see, however, 43]. In aging pulpal nerves the relative roles of pressure and of other factors (e.g. biological aging) in producing distal axonopathy and axon loss are naturally hard to assess. However, since the changes are so similar to those seen proximal to compressed or chronically severed nerves, it seems reasonable to assume that at least some of them represent reactions to pulpal space restrictions and to other age-related traumatic and irritating effects on the tooth.

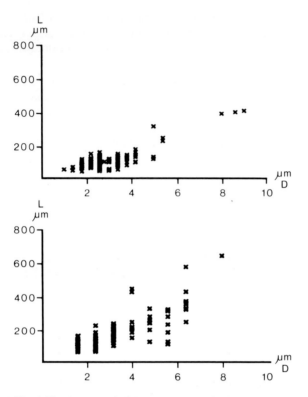

Fig. 6. The upper graph shows a representative example of the relation between inter-nodal length (L) and fibre diameter (D) of pulpal nerve fibres in the aging canine tooth of the cat. For comparison, the lower graph shows the relation L/D in young adult pulpal nerve fibres. From ref. [26, 27].

In old pulps, small groups of axons or bundles of collagen fibres are often surrounded by perineurium-like sheaths. Although present around pulpal stem axons in the IAN at all ages [30], such sheaths are not found in young adult pulps. In fact, the dental pulp was long considered as one of the few sites where axons lack a perineural investment [59], with the implication that, for example, toxins can easily reach the trigeminal gan-glion and the CNS from the pulp via the stem nerve endoneurium. How-ever, axons in old pulps are indeed invested by perineural sheaths which are formed from cells which initially resemble fibroblasts [cf. 75]. It has been suggested [80] that fibroblastic encirclement of Schwann cell bands with subsequent transformation to a perineurium-like sheath is a basic reaction to nerve injury. The appearance of perineural sheaths in old pulps may thus be a response to the age-related loss of axons.

Aging of Trigeminal Nerve Trunks that are Related to the Teeth

The axons which transmit impulses from the pulps and periodontal ligaments of the mandibular teeth run in the IAN. The mental branch of this nerve also conveys sensory information from the chin and lower lip [66]. Since the IAN enters the mandibular canal as a distinct nerve trunk, morphological age-related events are more easily followed here than in any of the numerous maxillary nerve branches supplying the dentition of the upper jaw. The pre- and postnatal maturation of IAN axons occurs in an orderly relation to the development of their peripheral field of innervation and to suckling and chewing [30–32]. It is noteworthy that neither the shedding of the primary mandibular teeth nor the formation of the permanent dentition structurally affects the IAN. However, in the old IAN, axonal and perineurial changes co-exist with signs of dental attrition or pathology. The axonal changes are of the same type that can be seen in the aging tooth pulp at apical levels: atrophic myelinated axons, Schwann cell extensions into axons (fig. 8) and features indicating axonal regeneration and/or remyelination. Degeneration of unmyelinated axons also seems to occur. Again, it is impossible to assess the roles of different factors, e.g. chronic disease, vascular changes, biological aging as such, or dental pathology producing these IAN nerve fibre alterations. However, senescent axonal injury is not found in the mental nerve [24], a branch which normally lacks dental nerve fibres [68]. This may be an indication that the IAN axonal changes are actually secondary to the gradual deterioration of the dentition in old age. Calculations show that although the total number of IAN axons in young and old cats appears to be similar, the percentage of unmyelinated fibres and the number of such axons per Schwann cell profile tend to be lower in old age [31]. This suggests that de novo myelination continues in this nerve into advanced age stages. It cannot be excluded, however, that a selective loss of unmyelinated axons may also contribute to these observations. Myelin sheath morphology of IAN axons in older individuals show some differences as compared to younger stages [32]. The maximum number of myelin lamellae surrounding individual axons increases with age, suggesting that ongoing myelination is a prolonged process, possibly extending over the entire life span. This fact, together with the gradual onset of senescent axonal atrophy, results in a less regular relation between myelin sheath thickness and axon size [cf. 47]. This is reflected in a much wider range of g-values (ratio of axon size to total fibre diameter) in old age. g-values of axons can be used to predict conduction properties of individual fibres [82]. They usually vary between 0.7 and 0.9 in peripheral nerves (including the young adult IAN) and this has been calculated to be

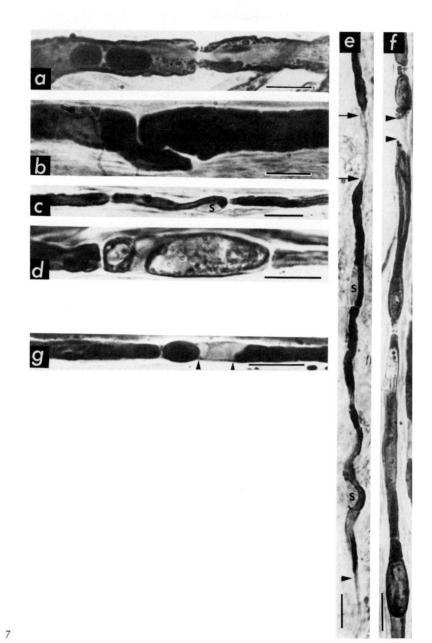

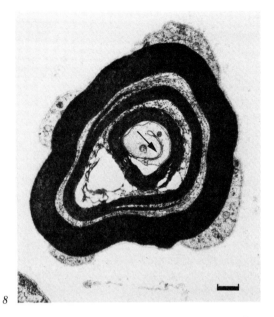

8

Fig. 8. Electron micrograph from the inferior alveolar nerve in an old (11 years) cat. A seemingly atrophic axon is surrounded by a thick myelin sheath subdivided into rings by cytoplasmic clefts. A Schwann cell expansion invaginates the axon (arrow). Scale bar 1 μm. From ref. [30].

Fig. 7. Photomicrographs depicting pulpal nerve fibres from aging cat canine teeth. From ref. [27]. All scale bars 10 μm. *a, b* Nodal-paranodal regions of two large axons. In *a*, some dark staining bodies are present in the left paranodal segment. In *b*, the node of Ranvier is partly covered by a large myelin fold. *c* An extremely short intercalated internode with the Schwann cell nucleus (asterisk) eccentrically situated. *d* An extremely short distorted internode. No Schwann cell nucleus is discernible. *e* Nerve fibre from the crown region. A wide node of Ranvier (between arrows) is followed by two short terminal internodes (asterisks at Schwann cell nuclei). The fibre then continues as an unmyelinated axon (arrowhead). *f* A nerve fibre with myelin ovoids and a segment (between arrowheads) devoid of myelin. *g* A nerve fibre with what appears to be a paranodal segment devoid of myelin (between arrowheads).

the range in which axon conduction is optimal [72; see further 79]. In old IAN, the g-values generally range between 0.3 and 0.7, suggesting that conduction in these axons may be different in senescence [cf. 16, 70, 77]. Internodal lengths in young and old IAN axons are, as expected, similar. An interesting finding in the old IAN is, however, the occurrence of short (100–150 μm) internodes appearing in succession on small axons. These internodes have probably developed on regenerated axons which may sprout as a response to axonal injury in teeth or periodontal tissues.

The axonal bundles in the IAN are surrounded by a perineurium which in old age tends to develop unusually thick basement membranes around the perineurial cells [30]. The reason for this is unclear; this feature does not seem to have been observed in nerves in other regions during aging. However, it appears to be present in some pathological states. Thus, thickened basement membranes are found along perineurial cells in Fabry's disease [10] and in diabetes mellitus [41]. Some findings indicate that such a thickening may be correlated to myelinated axon loss [41]. Its appearance in the old IAN could thus be related to dental axon injury and loss.

Structural Alterations of Dental Axons as Related to Possible Functional Changes in Senescence

As seen from the foregoing text, aging of permanent pulpal nerves involves at least two striking components: (1) disease and loss of terminal axon branches, and (2) stem nerve fibre changes which may be secondary to this process. Pulpal axon loss in senescence parallels clinical findings of reduced sensitivity to electrical pulpal stimulation in aging subjects [55]. This may, however, also reflect changes in nerve fibre function due to axonal remodelling in the terminal area after, e.g. secondary dentine formation [13]. De- and regenerative myelin sheath remodelling, affecting fibre conduction properties, may also be involved. It should be remembered, though, that responses to clinical tooth pulp stimuli could be different due to psychological changes in pain perception with age [83].

In addition to effects on 'normal' pulpal pain transmission, some of the events mentioned here might yield nerve fibres with pathologically increased excitability. Normal stem nerves are virtually indifferent to mechanical stimuli. However, peripheral nerves that are experimentally demyelinated become very mechanosensitive, even when subjected to very light mechanical stimuli [63]. The ability of the pathological, de-myelinated fibre to generate impulse activity at such ectopic sites could be of interest when searching for aetiological factors related to chronic pain states in the trigeminal area. On the basis of physiological findings it has been suggested that focal demyelination in the trigeminal root may cause pain syndromes in the trigeminal system [12]. Demyelination in peripheral branches as a result of senescent tooth pulp axon injury and loss could hypothetically also be a source of abnormal pain.

Ectopic activity and abnormal mechanosensitivity develop not only after demyelination. They are also prominent in neuromas, the peripheral ends of nerves in which regeneration after injury is hindered [15]. With the loss of pulpal terminal nerve fibres in old age, due to pulpal pathology or tooth loss, a number of pulpal stem fibres probably react with end sprouting and attempts at regeneration; we know that at least the young adult IAN has a very strong regenerative capacity [25]. IAN sprouts, devoid of pulpal and/or periodontal targets, may, in a frustrated regenerative attempt, then form small neuromas in the skin or the alveolar/buccal mucosa. As early as 1936, Bradlaw [11] found evidence of regeneration of severed apical nerves after tooth extractions. He suggested that this might explain neuralgia following multiple extractions. In a light microscopical study, alveolar mucosa biopsies from old edentulous patients were found to contain abnormal masses of nerve tissue [49]. This was especially evident in areas which were clinically established as being hypersensitive ('trigger spots'). Later studies have confirmed that neuralgia in oral regions often coexists with deterioration of the dentition [52, 65]. In fact, one author states that removal of teeth or pulpectomy is the most frequent etiological factor in the history of older (>50 years) patients with painful oral traumatic neuromas [64].The clinical consequences of these processes may be great suffering from pain; in addition, conditions may be aggravated by the fact that patients with these problems often are unable to wear dentures, since these devices provoke pain.

The progressive tooth pulp pathology and tooth loss in old age may induce changes in peripheral nerve segments which may, in some instances, result in pain syndromes. In addition to the possible peripheral sources of pain, transmission from dental pulps and oral tissues may be affected by age-related changes in the other structures in the trigeminal system which are associated with oral and dental targets. In the trigeminal ganglion of the mouse, aging seems to involve an increase in vacuolar cell degeneration [3]; the possible functional consequences of this are not clear. Furthermore, since tooth pulp removal and tooth extractions in young adult cats result in transganglionic changes in the spinal trigeminal nucleus [34, 81], central remodelling is also likely to occur after senescent tooth pulp pathology and tooth loss. The morphology and function in old age of the CNS trigeminal pathways related to tooth pulp pain and proprioception remain challenging fields for future investigations.

Summary

The life history of permanent tooth pulp axons can be described as composed of three phases. Initial ingrowth of axons takes place shortly before and during root resorption and pulpal axon degeneration in the primary teeth. This is concomitant with mineralization and root formation. Axon ingrowth and maturation then continues past eruption and is completed when the tooth is functionally mature and the apical foramen closes. After this, a short relatively stable stage occurs with no major changes in the pulpal innervation. However, as the individual grows older and the dentition begins to show regressive changes, a protracted phase involving axonal changes and axon loss follows. Some teeth may become completely denervated. It seems likely that some of the nerve fibre alterations represent reactions to pulpal space restrictions and to other age-related traumatic and irritating effects on the tooth. In nerve trunks which supply the teeth with sensory axons, old-age axonal and perineurial changes also occur. Since these are of a type that typically occur proximal to neurotomies, they are probably secondary to the deterioration of the permanent dentition. Degeneration and loss of pulpal nerve fibres may affect transmission from pulpal structures, resulting in increased thresholds to pain stimuli. In addition, myelin sheath changes and terminal axon remodelling subsequent to age-related dental axon injury could be sources of abnormal pain in the oral region.

Acknowledgements

Much of our own works cited here were done in collaboration with Dr. Claes Hildebrand, to whom grateful thanks are extended. These studies were supported by grants from the Swedish Medical Research Council (Project No. 3761), Karolinska Institutet, and the Swedish Dental Association. Many thanks to Prof. Marshall Devor for comments on the manuscript, and for providing facilities when preparing this chapter during a sabbatical at Hebrew University, Jerusalem. Thanks also to Dr. Izak Paul for valuable suggestions.

References

1 Aitken, J. T.; Thomas, P. K.: Retrograde changes in fibre size following nerve section. J. Anat. 96: 121–129 (1962).
2 Alexander, S. A.; Swerdloff, M.: Mucopolysaccharidase activity during human deciduous root resorption. Archs oral Biol. 24: 735–738 (1979).
3 Andrew, W.: Cytological changes in senility in the trigeminal ganglion, spinal cord and brain of the mouse. J. Anat. 75: 406–418 (1941).
4 Azaz, B.; Michaeli, Y.; Nitzan, D.: Aging of tissues of the roots of nonfunctional human teeth (impacted canines). Oral Surg. oral Med. oral Path. 43: 572–578 (1977).
5 Bennett, C. G.; Kelln, E. E.; Biddington, W. R.: Age changes of the vascular pattern of the human dental pulp. Archs oral Biol. 10: 995–998 (1965).
6 Bernick, S.: Age changes in the nerves of molar teeth of rats. Anat. Rec. 143: 121–126 (1962).
7 Bernick, S.: Effect of aging on the nerve supply to human teeth. J. dent. Res. 46: 544 (1967).
8 Bernick, S.: This volume.

9   Bernick, S.; Nedelman, C.: Effect of aging on the human pulp. J. Endodont. *1:* 88–94 (1975).

10 Bischoff, A.: Peripheral nervous system; in Bischoff, Ultrastructure of the peripheral nervous system and sense organs, pp. 5–172 (Thieme, Stuttgart 1970).

11 Bradlaw, R.: The innervation of teeth. Proc. R. soc. Med. *32:* 1040–1053 (1936).

12 Burchiel, K. J.: Ectopic impulse generation in focally demyelinated trigeminal nerve. Exp Neurol. *69:* 423–429 (1980).

13 Byers, M. R.: Development of sensory innervation in dentin. J. comp. Neurol. *191:* 413–427 (1980).

14 Byers, M. R.: Dental sensory receptors. Int. Rev. Neurobiol. *25:* 39–94 (1984).

15 Devor, M.: Nerve pathophysiology and mechanisms of pain in causalgia. J. autonom. nerv. Syst. *7:* 371–384 (1983).

16 Dorfman, L. J.; Bosley, T. M.: Age-related changes in peripheral and central nerve conduction in man. Neurology, Minncap. *29:* 38–44 (1979).

17 Dyck, P. J.; Nukada, H.; Lais, A. C.; Karnes, J. L.: Permanent axotomy: a model of chronic neuronal degeneration preceded by axonal atrophy, myelin remodeling and degeneration; in Dyck, Thomas, Lambert, Bunge, Peripheral neuropathy; 2nd ed. pp. 760–870 (Saunders, Philadelphia 1984).

18 Dyck, P. J.; Karnes, J. L.; Lais, A.; Lofgren, E. P.; Stevens, J. C.: Pathologic alterations of the peripheral nervous system of humans; in Dyck, Thomas, Lambert, Bunge, Peripheral neuropathy; 2nd ed., pp. 760–870 (Saunders, Philadelphia 1984).

19 Edwall, L.: Personal communication.

20 Erdelyi, G.; Fried, K.; Hildebrand, C.: Nerve growth to tooth buds after homotopic or heterotopic autotransplantation. Dev. Brain Res. (in press).

21 Fernhead, R. W.: The neurohistology of human dentine. Proc. R. Soc. Med. *54:* 877–884 (1961).

22 Fernhead, R. W.: Innervation of dental tissues; in Miles, Structure and chemical organization of teeth, vol. 1, pp. 247–281 (Academic Press, New York 1967).

23 Fried, K.: Development, degeneration and regeneration of nerve fibres in the feline inferior alveolar nerve and mandibular incisor pulps. Acta physiol. scand. suppl. 504, pp. 1–28 (1982).

24 Fried, K.: Structural development of the feline mental nerve. Anat. Rec. *210:* 347–355 (1984).

25 Fried, K.: Erdelyi, G.: Inferior alveolar nerve regeneration and incisor pulpal reinnervation following intramandibular neurotomy in the cat. Brain Res. *244:* 259–268 (1982).

26 Fried, K.; Erdelyi, G.: Short internodal lengths of canine tooth pulp axons in the young adult cat. Brain Res. *303:* 141–145 (1984).

27 Fried, K.; Erdelyi, G.: Changes with age in canine tooth pulp-nerve fibres of the cat. Archs oral Biol *29:* 581–585 (1984).

28 Fried, K.; Hildebrand, C.: Development, growth and degeneration of pulpal axons in feline primary incisors. J. comp. Neurol. *203:* 37–51 (1981).

29 Fried, K.; Hildebrand, C.: Pulpal axons in developing, mature and aging feline permanent incisors. A study by electron microscopy. J. comp. Neurol. *203:* 23–26 (1981).

30 Fried, K.; Hildebrand, C.: Qualitative structural development of the feline inferior alveolar nerve. J. Anat. *134:* 517–531 (1982).

31 Fried, K.; Hildebrand, C.: Axon number and size distribution in the developing feline inferior alveolar nerve. J. neurol. Sci. *53:* 169–180 (1982).

32 Fried, K.; Hildebrand, C.; Erdelyi, G.: Myelin sheath thickness and internodal length of nerve fibres in the developing feline inferior alveolar nerve. J. neurol. Sci. *54:* 47–57 (1982).

33 Fulling, H. J.; Andreasen, J. O.: Influence of maturation status and tooth type of permanent teeth upon electrometric and thermal pulp testing. Scand. J. dent. Res. *84:* 286–290 (1976).

34 Gobel, S.; Binck, J. M.: Degenerative changes in primary trigeminal axons and in neurons in nucleus caudalis following tooth pulp extirpations in the cat. Brain Res. *132:* 347–354 (1977).

35 Grover-Johnson, N.; Spencer, P. S.: Peripheral nerve abnormalities in aging rats. J. Neuropath. exp. Neurol. *40:* 155–165 (1981).

36 Gunji, T.: Morphological research on the sensitivity of dentin. Arch. Histol. Jap. *45:* 45–67 (1982).

37 Gunji, T.; Gunji, K.; Hoshino, M.; Takeuchi, K.; Kobayashi, S.: Morphological change of pulpal nerves with advancing years. Jap. J. oral Biol. *25:* 503–529 (1983).

38 Johnsen, D. C.: Innervation of teeth: qualitative, quantitative and developmental assessment. J. dent. Res. *64: spec. iss.*, pp. 555–563 (1985).

39 Johnsen, D. C.; Harshbarger, J.; Rymer, H. D.: Quantitative assessment of neural development in human premolars. Anat. Rec. *205:* 421–429 (1983).

40 Johnsen, D. C.; Karlsson, U. L.: Electron microscopic quantitations of feline primary and permanent incisor innervation. Archs oral Biol. *19:* 671–678 (1974).

41 Johnson, P. C.: Thickening of the human dorsal root ganglion perineurial cell basement membrane in diabetes mellitus. Muscle Nerve *6:* 561–565 (1983).

42 Ketterl, W.: Age-induced changes in the teeth and their attachment apparatus. Int. dent. J. *33:* 262–271 (1983).

43 King, R. H. M.; Thomas, P. K.: Ultrastructural changes in peripheral nerve with ageing. 9th Meet. of Swiss Neuropathologists with International Participation, St. Moritz 1982.

44 Klein, H.: Pulp responses to an electric pulp stimulator in the developing permanent anterior dentition. J. dent. Child. *45:* 199–202 (1978).

45 Kohari, S.; Bona, K.: Vergleichende elektronenmikroskopische Untersuchungen von Zahnschmelz and Dentin bei Individuen verschiedenen Alters. Dt. zahnärtzl. Z. *15:* 1009–1020 (1960).

46 Korthals, J. K.; Wisniewski, H. M.: Peripheral nerve ischemia. 1. Experimental model. J. neurol. Sci. *24:* 65–76 (1975).

47 Lascelles, R. G.; Thomas, P. K.: Changes due to age in internodal length in the sural nerve in man. J. Neurol. Neurosurg. Psychiat. *29:* 40–44 (1966).

48 Lovasi, Z.; Boros, S.; Banoczy, J.; Sobkowiak, E. M.: Histologische Untersuchung der Zahnpulpa von kariesfreien, periodontal erkrankten Zähnen. Zahn-, Mund-Kieferheilkd. *72:* 17–23 (1984).

49 Marsland, E. A.; Fox, E. C.: Some abnormalities in the nerve supply of the oral mucosa. Proc. R. Soc. Med. *51:* 951–956 (1958).

50 Mendis, B. R. R. M.; Darling, A. I.: Distribution with age and attrition of peritubular dentin in the crowns of human teeth. Archs oral Biol. *24:* 131–139 (1979).

51 Miles, A. E. W.: Ageing in the teeth and oral tissues; in Bourne, Structural aspects of ageing, pp. 352–397 (Pitman, London 1961).

52 Mitchell, R. G.: Pre-trigeminal neuralgia. Br. dent. J. *149:* 1–4 (1980).

53 Moore, G. E.: Age changes occurring in the teeth. J. forens. Sci. Soc. *10:* 179–180 (1970).

54 Morris, J. H.; Hudson, A. R.; Weddell, G.: A study of degeneration and regeneration in the divided rat sciatic nerve based on electron microscopy. III. Changes in the axons of the proximal stump. Z. Zellforsch. *124:* 131–164 (1972).

55 Mumford, J. M.: Pain perception threshold and adaptation of normal human teeth. Arch oral Biol. *10:* 957–968 (1965).

56 Obst, T.: Über das Endgebiet des Perinurium an der Zahnnerven der Ratte. Z. Zel-
    lforsch. *114:* 515–531 (1971).
57 Ochoa, J.; Fowler, T. J.; Gilliatt, R. W.: Anatomical changes in peripheral nerves
    compressed by a pneumatic torniquet. J. Anat. *113:* 433–455 (1972).
58 Ochoa, J.; Mair, W. G. P.: The normal sural nerve in man. II. Changes in the axons
    and Schwann cells due to ageing. Acta neuropath. *13:* 217–239 (1969).
59 Olsson, Y.: Vascular permeability in the peripheral nervous system; in Dyck, Thomas,
    Lambert, Peripheral neuropathy, vol. 1, pp. 190–200 (Saunders, Philadelphia 1975).
60 Pearson, A. A.: The relation of ingrowing nerve fibres to developing tooth buds in
    human embroys. J. Anat. *181:* 446 (1974).
61 Pearson, A. A.: The early innervation of developing deciduous teeth. J. Anat. *123:*
    563–577 (1977).
62 Quigley, M. B.: Functional and geriatric changes of the human pulp. Oral Surg. oral
    Med. oral Pathol. *32:* 795–806 (1971).
63 Rasminsky, M.: Ectopic impulse generation in pathological nerve fibres. Trends
    Neurosci. *6:* 388–390 (1983).
64 Rasmussen, O. C.: Painful traumatic neuromas in the oral cavity. Oral Surg. oral Med.
    oral Path. *49:* 191–195 (1980).
65 Ratner, E. J.; Person, P.; Kleinman, D. J.; Shklar, G.; Socransky, S. S.: Jawbone cavi-
    ties and trigeminal and atypical facial neuralgias. Oral Surg. oral Med. oral Path. *48:*
    3–20 (1979).
66 Robinson, P. P.: The course, relations and distribution of the inferior alveolar nerve in
    the cat. Anat. Rec. *195:* 265–272 (1979).
67 Robinson, P. P.: Reinnervation of teeth, mucous membrane and skin following section
    of the inferior alveolar nerve in the cat. Brain Res. *220:* 241–253 (1981).
68 Robinson, P. P.: An electrophysiological study of the pathways of pulpal nerves from
    mandibular teeth in the cat. Archs oral Biol. *25:* 825–829 (1980).
69 Samorajski, T.: Age differences in the morphology of posterior tibial nerves of mice.
    J. comp. Neurol. *157:* 439–452 (1974).
70 Sato. A.; Sato, Y.; Suzuki, H.: Aging effects on conduction velocities of myelinated
    and unmyelinated fibres of peripheral nerves. Neurosci. Lett. *53:* 15–20 (1985).
71 Sharma, A. K.; Bajada, S.; Thomas, P. K.: Age changes in the tibial and plantar
    nerves of the rat. J. Anat. *130:* 417–428 (1980).
72 Smith, R. S.; Koles, Z. J.: Myelinated nerve fibers – computed effect of myelin sheath
    thickness on conduction velocity. Am. J. Physiol. *219:* 1256–1258 (1970).
73 Spencer, P. S.; Thomas, P. K.: Ultrastructural studies of the dying-back process. II.
    The sequestration and removal by Schwann cells and oligodendrocytes of organelles
    from normal and diseased axons. J. Neurocytol. *3:* 763–783 (1974).
74 Takagi, M.: Studies on the dental innervation of tooth germs in the developmental
    stage. J. Osaka Dent. Univ. *1:* 50–64 (1967).
75 Thomas, P. K.; Bhagat, S.: The effect of extraction of the intrafascicular contents of
    peripheral nerve trunks of perineurial structure. Acta neuropath. *43:* 135–141 (1978).
76 Thomas, P. K.; King, R. H. M.; Sharma, A. K.: Changes with age in the peripheral
    nerves of the rat. An ultrastructural study. Acta neuropath. *52:* 1–6 (1980).
77 Tohgi, H.; Tsukagoshi, H.; Toyokura, Y.: Quantitative changes with age in normal
    sural nerves. Acta neuropath. *38:* 213–220 (1977).
78 Tomes, C. S.: A manual of dental anatomy; 3rd ed. (Churchill, London 1889).
79 Waxman, S. G.: Variations in axonal morphology; in Waxman, Physiology and patho-
    biology of axons, pp. 169–190 (Raven Press, New York 1978).
80 Weinberg, H. J.; Spencer, P. S.: The fate of Schwann cells isolated from axonal con-
    tact. J. Neurocytol. *7:* 555–569 (1979).

81 Westrum, L. E.; Canfield, R. C.; Black, R. G.: Transganglionic degeneration in the spinal trigeminal nucleus following removal of tooth pulps in adult cats. Brain Res. *101:* 137–140 (1976).

82 Williams, P. L.; Wendell-Smith, C. P.: Some additional parametric variations between peripheral nerve fibre populations. J. Anat. *109:* 505–526 (1971).

83 Woodrow, K. M.; Friedman, G. D.; Siegelaub, A. B.; Collen, M. F.: Pain tolerance: differences according to age, sex and race; in Weisenberg, Pain, clinical and experimental perspectives, pp. 133–140 (Mosby, St. Louis 1975).

84 Ziliken, F.: Biologie des Alterns; in Sauerwein, Gerontostomatologie, pp. 28–60 (Thieme, Stuttgart 1981).

K. Fried, DDS, PhD, Department of Anatomy, Karolinska Institutet,
POB 60 400, S-104 01 Stockholm 60 (Sweden)

Front. oral Physiol., vol. 6, pp. 85–95 (Karger, Basel 1987)

Collagen in Aging Bone of the Jaw

H. Shikata[a], N. Utsumi[a], D. Fujimoto[b]

[a] Department of Oral Pathology, Josai Dental University, Sakado, Saitama; and
[b] Department of Agricultural chemistry, Tokyo Noko University, Fuchu, Tokyo, Japan

Introduction

Bone undergoes morphological and physiological changes during an animal's life time. The differences in physical and mechanical properties of bone at different stages of development are affected by, for example, the extent of mineralization, but recent work in our laboratory also suggests that chemical changes in bone protein occur during maturation or aging.

Collagen, the most abundant protein in man and animals, accounts for about 90% of the non-mineralized content of bone [31]. To date, 11 genetically distinct types of collagen have been assigned Roman numerals by their discoverers or their characterizers [2]. Type I collagen is the collagen found in bone. It has a rod-like molecule about 300 nm in length and is constructed from three polypeptide chains wound into a triple helix and each molecule contains rather short non-helical peptides at each end (N-terminus and C-terminus), the telopeptides, which are sites of cross-linking. In the extracellular matrix, type I collagen assembles into multi-unit structures called fibrils that provide the structural framework of bone. Fibril bundles are then formed to the point where gross fibers may be identified in bone and other tissues.

Cross-linking of collagen has received a great deal of attention because of its role in determining the properties of fibrils. It is generally accepted that the collagen fiber increases in stability with aging, and that this maturation or aging process is related to the content and/or chemical nature of the cross-links. For example, old collagen is less suspectible to digestion by proteolytic enzymes and shows a decreased ability to swell in several solvents. These changes are due to the formation of cross-links [15]. In this section, we should like to consider present knowledge on age-related changes of cross-links in collagen of the mandibular or maxillary bones.

Cross-Linking of Collagen

To develop the necessary tensile strength, the collagen fibril must acquire intermolecular cross-links. Cross-linking is initiated by the oxidative deamination of the ε-amino groups of specific lysyl and hydroxylysyl residues near the end of the collagen molecules to produce reactive aldehydes. Oxidative deamination is catalyzed by the enzyme lysyl oxidase. After the aldehyde groups are generated by lysyl oxidase, Schiff bases are formed as intermolecular cross-links in collagen. The initially formed aldimine cross-link is unstable and hydroxylysine-containing cross-links are converted to the more stable keto form by an Amadori rearrangement. Both the aldimine and the keto forms of the cross-links are borohydride reducible [32]. Most of these cross-links are unstable to acid hydrolysis and can be isolated only after reduction with sodium borohydride and thereafter called 'reducible cross-links' [32]. It has been shown that reducible cross-links are found in large quantities at very young ages and, in newly synthesized collagen. Moreover, they graduately disappear toward maturity [1, 3]. It has been suggested that these cross-links are replaced by more complex non-reducible cross-links during maturation. However, the structures of the non-reducible and acid stable cross-links, which are responsible for the aging process, have proved to be elusive for a long time. Our laboratory has isolated several non-reducible cross-linking amino acids from connective tissues [4, 7].

Pyridinoline, 'Mature' Cross-Linking Amino Acid

Collagen is known to contain visibly fluorescent materials and the concentration of these materials increases with age [15]. However, the chemical nature of these materials has not been elucidated. We isolated the fluorescent and ninhydrin-positive materials from acid hydrolysates of bovine Achilles tendon collagen [4, 5]. The structure shown in figure 1 suggests that this fluorescent material is a trifunctional cross-link. It is a 3-hydroxypyridinium derivative with 3 amino and 3 carboxyl groups and was therefore termed 'pyridinoline'.

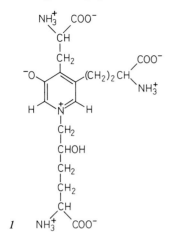

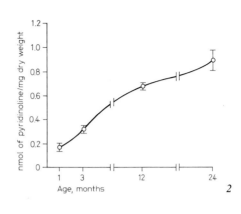

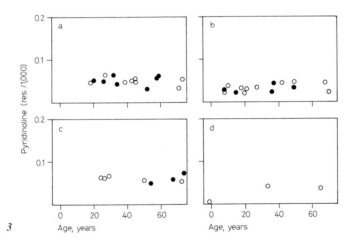

Fig. 1. Structure of pyridinoline.

Fig. 2. Age-related changes in the content of pyridinoline in rat mandibular bone.

Fig. 3. Age-related changes in human bone. Reproduced with permission from ref. [13]. *a* Mandibula; *b* Maxilla; *c* Femur; *d* rib. ○ = Male; ● = female.

Age-Related Changes in the Content of Pyridinoline

Pyridinoline is acid-stable and can be isolated without reduction: it is therefore considered to be a 'mature' cross-link. Pyridinoline has been reported to be more abundant in mature connective tissues than in growing or young tissues [22]. Moreover, the synthesis of pyridinoline cross-links from lysyl residues has been demonstrated in vitro using ^{14}C-lysine-labelled collagen and purified lysyl oxidase [29].

The age-related changes in the pyridinoline content in the collagen of mandibular or maxillary bone have been investigated [27]. The results are shown in figures 2 and 3. The pyridinoline content in young rats was very low but it increased markedly with growth of the animals and aging. This marked increase was found by the time the animal reached physiological maturity, i.e. about 6 months of age. After reaching maturity, the pyridinoline content continued to increased slowly with aging. In man, the pyridinoline content increased maximally during puberty, and then remained constant throughout life (fig. 3.). No significant difference in pyridinoline content was found between mandibular and maxillary bone collagen. Age-related changes of pyridinoline in human dentine collagen showed a similar pattern to those of human mandibular and maxillary bone collagen (fig. 4). Similar age-related changes in the content of pyridinoline have been found in other connective tissues [13]. The increase of pyridinoline content appears to be concomitant with decrease in the content of reducible cross-links [1] and with increase in mechanical strength of collagen fibril [24]. It is therefore likely that pyridinoline is related to the maturation of collagen.

The fact that the pyridinoline content in cartilage collagen decreases with age after maturity [22] is of interest in relation to senile changes in tissue. To explain why the pyridinoline content does not increase markedly after maturity, 'senescent' cross-links which increase with age after maturity have been postulated. Recently, a candidate for the senescent cross-links which are involved in senile changes of connective tissues has been discovered.

Histidinoalanine, 'Senescent' Cross-Linking Amino Acid

The cross-link which may be involved in senile changes is identified as histidinoalanine or N^{τ}-(2-aminocarboxymethyl)histidine [7]. As shown in figure 5, it is a bifunctional cross-linking amino acid and is a cross-link not derived from lysine and hydroxylysine. Its lineage differs from that of reducible cross-links and pyridinoline. Histidinoalanine was first discov-

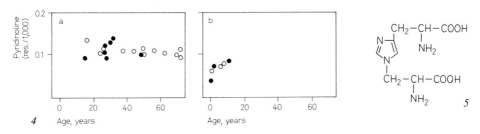

Fig. 4. Age-related changes in the content of pyridinoline in human dentine. Reproduced with permission from ref. [13]. *a* Permanent; *b* deciduous. ○ = Male; ● = female.

Fig. 5. Structure of histidinoalanine.

ered in human dentine collagen [7] and subsequently found in proteins of various connective tissues [8, 9]. It is abundant in costal cartilage and aorta where its concentration increases linearly with age [8, 9]. It is increasingly being accepted that this cross-link is associated with collagen. The age-related changes in the histidinoalanine content of rat mandibular bone are described below [27].

Age-Related Changes in the Content of Histidinoalanine of Rat Mandibular Bone

As shown in figure 6, this cross-link is less abundant in young animals but, after maturity, it becomes significantly more abundant with age. Thus, it is clear that histidinoalanine is associated with the senile changes of rat mandibular bone. In the light of other findings, histidinoalanine can be said to be present generally in aged connective tissues. Therefore, it is proposed that this cross-link is a 'senescent cross-link'. It is so far not known whether this cross-link is present in the collagen of mandibular bone and/or other bones.

Histidinoalanine is probably formed by interaction of a histidine residue in one peptide chain with a serine (or a cysteine) residue in another peptide chain. The reaction is probably non-enzymic and may proceed slowly under physiological conditions.

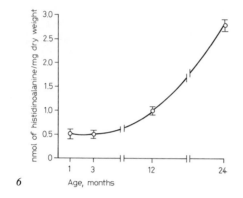

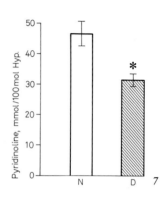

6

7

Fig. 6. Age-related changes in the content of histidinoalanine in rat mandibular bone. Reproduced with permission from ref. [27].

Fig. 7. Pyridinoline content in mandibular bone from normal (N) and diabetic (D) groups. Reproduced with permission from ref. [26]. Each column shows the mean ± SE of 6 animals. *p < 0.01 vs normal (Student's t-test).

Accelerating Aging of Collagen by Maillard Reaction or Non-Enzymatic Browning

It is known that glycosylation and cross-linking occur in food proteins that are stored in the presence of sugars, probably due to a Maillard reaction, otherwise known as non-enzymatic browning [14, 23]. For example, glucose is bound non-enzymatically to free amino groups of proteins. The products of the reactions then undergo Amadori rearrangement and with time dehydrate to form fluorescent compounds. Recently, it has been proposed that a Maillard reaction occurs in collagen [10, 20, 21], particularly in diabetes mellitus. Collagen from individuals with diabetes is less soluble and has increased mechanical stiffness, and increased thermal stability, suggesting that increased cross-link formation has occurred. Therefore, diabetes can be considered to accelerate the aging of collagen.

Three factors responsible for these age- and diabetes-related effects have been postulated. One of them is that the increased cross-linking of collagen may be due to the increase of lysyl-oxidase-dependant or pyridinoline cross-links. Increased levels of lysyl oxidase activity have been observed in diabetic tissues [18]. However, it has been reported that no

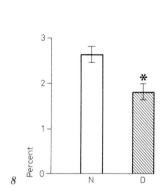

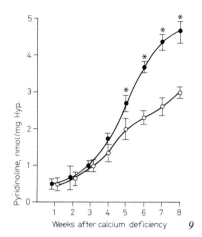

Fig. 8. Ratio of collagen digestibility by pepsin. Reproduced with permission from ref. [26]. Each column shows the mean ± SE of 6 animals. *p < 0.01 vs normal control.

Fig. 9. Changes in pyridinoline content of normal and calcium-deficient rat mandibular bone. Reproduced with permission from ref. [28]. Each point shows the mean ± SE of 6 animals. ○ = Control; ● = calcium deficiency. *p < 0.01 vs control animals.

significant difference in the amounts of reducible cross-links was found between normal and diabetic tissues [17]. The second possibility is that histidinoalanine is involved in cross-link abnormality. The third is that the Maillard reaction may play a role in the formation of increased cross-linking of collagen. Collagen contains many lysyl and hydroxylyslyl residues with free amino groups and seems to be exposed to ambient levels of extracellular glucose so that it may be particular vulnerable to such reactions. We examined the effect of experimentally induced diabetes on the content of pyridinoline and histidinoalanine cross-links in rat mandibular bone [26]. Two-month-old male Wistar rats weighing approximately 240g were used in this study. Diabetes was induced by intravenous injection of 70mg/kg body weight of streptozotocin. Twenty-one days after the injection, the mandibular bone was studied for its content of pyridinoline and histidinoalanine, and the digestibility of its collagen by pepsin.

As shown in figures 7 and 8, the pyridinoline content of mandibular bone collagen and its solubility by pepsin were significantly decreased in diabetic animals. However, no significant difference of histidinoalanine content was found between normal and diabetic animals (data not shown). These results suggested that maturation of collagen was inhibited, although other experiments showed that collagen stability was increased by diabetes. It is reasonable to speculate that the increased stability to pepsin is due to increased cross-linking as a result of a Maillard reaction. This idea was recently supported by Monnier [21] who reported that the Maillard reaction may impair cross-link formation in newly synthesized collagen, but it may accelerate cross-link formation in mature collagen. However, Maillard reaction products have been detected in increased amount in collagen from aged and/or diabetic individuals [10, 20, 21], suggesting that the Maillard reaction may be an important factor in the aging process of collagen.

The precise structure and character of Maillard reaction products in collagen molecules is not yet known in detail. Also, nothing is known about the Maillard reaction of mandibular or maxillary bone collagen. We expect that further study of non-enzymic cross-linking processes will improve our understanding of age- and diabetes-related changes of collagen.

Possible Role of Collagen Cross-Linking in Mineralization of Bone

Bone collagen is generally known to be resistant to solubilization and swelling, indicating that it is highly cross-linked. One question about cross-linking of bone collagen is: 'What is the role of collagen cross-linking in mineralization?' A few experimental studies have attempted to determining whether cross-link formation is related to the mineralization of bone. Studies with experimentally induced vitamin D- and phosphorus-deficient animals have demonstrated that pyridinoline exists exclusively in collagen of non-mineralized bone [6, 33, 34], but is almost absent in the mineralized bone [19]. Although the relationship between these pathological conditions and the mechanism for the increasing pyridinoline formation is unclear, pyridinoline may prevent the entrance of calcium ions into collagen fibrils and the subsequent formation of hydroxyapatite.

It is also interesting that in human atherosclerotic aortas a marked increase of histidinoalanine content was found in the 'mineralized' portions of calcified lesions [11]. Pyridinoline content was also increased but to a lesser extent [11]. Recently, high concentrations of histidinoalanine have been found within a phosphoprotein; this protein is considered to bind calcium and serve as the transporter of calcium ions in the tissue [16, 25]. These observations tentatively suggest that cross-linking may have a role in mineralization. We examined the influence of mineralization on pyridinoline and histidinoalanine formation in mandibular bone using calcium-deficient rats [28]. Four-week-old male Wistar rats were raised for 8 weeks on calcium-deficient diets. Calcium deficiency caused decreases of serum and bone calcium levels as well as growth retardation at 4 weeks after the start of experiment (data not shown). In contrast, the content of pyridinoline in the mandibular bone was observed to increase with the growth of the animals (fig. 9), whereas histidinoalanine content remained the same (data not shown).

These results suggest that pyridinoline synthesis is impaired by mineralization, but histidinoalanine synthesis is unrelated to the mineralization of bone. We do not know the precise effect of calcium-deficiency on changes in bone remodelling and in causing increased pyridinoline synthesis. However, these data are consistent with the previous suggestion. Further study is necessary to determine the physiological function of cross-linking in the mineralization of bone. More extensive evidence may also provide us with a better understanding of many diseases in which abnormal mineralization occurs.

Conclusion

The 'three-phase cross-links' hypothesis first proposed by Fujimoto [12] to describe the equilibrium between immature, mature and senescent cross-links can be used to study the common aging of connective tissue proteins. Recent studies on the aging of collagen in several tissues have provided support for this hypothesis [21, 27].

As described above, the content of cross-links varies with animal species, in different tissues, and also with age. Because humans have a much longer life span than experimental animals, study of human tissues is much more likely to provide evidence about mature and senescent cross-links. Since collagen has a very slow turnover rate, it may be predisposed to non-enzymic cross-linking reactions such as histidinoalanine formation or the Maillard reaction. These non-enzymic cross-linking reactions probably occur in aged collagen and other connective tissue proteins. The accumulation of these cross-links may change the chemical or physical properties of collagen.

Finally, we believe that cross-links other than those discussed here will probably be found to be associated with the aging process of connective tissue proteins. The accumulating knowledge about cross-links will enable us to expand to the 'three-phase cross-links' hypothesis. Understanding of the process of aging of collagen in the oral tissues will progress more quickly as more information about cross-links in other connective tissues is gathered.

Acknowledgement

The authors wish to thank Drs. M. Hiramatsu, Department of Dental Pharmacology, Josai Dental University, and K. E. Kadler, Department of Biochemistry, Jefferson Medical College, for their helpful suggestions. The research work was supported in part by Grants-in-Aid from the Ministry of Education, Science and Culture, Japan.

References

1   Bailey, A. J.; Shimokomaki, M. S.: Age-related changes in the reducible cross-links in collagen. FEBS Lett. *16:* 86–89 (1971).

2   Cheah, K. S. E.: Collagen genes and inherited connective tissue disease. Biochem. J. *229:* 287–303 (1985).

3   Fujii, K.; Tanzer, M. L.: Age-related changes in the reducible crosslinks of human tendon collagen. FEBS Lett. *43:* 300–302 (1974).

4   Fujimoto, D.; Akiba, K.; Nakamura, N.: Isolation and characterization of a fluorescent material from bovine Achilles tendon collagen. Biochem. biophys. Res. Commun. *76:* 1124–1128 (1977).

5   Fujimoto, D.; Moriguchi, T.; Ishida, T.; Hayashi, H.: The structure of pyridinoline, a collagen crosslink. Biochem. biophys. Res. Commun. *54:* 52–57 (1978).

6   Fujimoto, D.; Fujie, M.; Abe, E.; Suda, T.: Effect of vitamin D on the content of the stable crosslinks, pyridinoline, in chick bone collagen. Biochem. biophys. Res. Commun. *91:* 24–28 (1979).

7   Fujimoto, D.; Hirama, M.; Iwashita, T.: Histidinoalanine, a new crosslinking amino acid, in calcified tissue collagen. Biochem. biophys. Res. Commun. *104:* 1102–1106 (1982).

8   Fujimoto, D.: Aging and crosslinking in human aorta. Biochem. biophys. Res. Commum. *109:* 1264–1269 (1982).

9   Fujimoto, D.: Aging of human connective tissue. Increase in the content of a crosslinking amino acid, histidinoalanine. Biochem. int. *5:* 743–746 (1982).

10 Fujimoto, D.: Human tendon collagen: aging and crosslinking. Biomed. Res. 279–282 (1984).

11 Fujimoto, D.; Yu, S. Y.: Elevation of histidinoalanine in calcified human aortas. Biochem. int. *8:* 553–560 (1984).

12 Fujimoto, D.: What causes aging? in Fujimoto, (Kodansha, Tokyo 1984).

13 Fujimoto, D.: Pyridinoline, a new crosslink of collagen and its change in aging; in Robert, Murata, Nagai, Degenerative diseases of connective tissue and aging, pp. 35–45 (Kodansha, Tokyo 1985).

14 Keeney, M.; Bassette, R.: Detection of intermediate compounds in the early stages of browning reaction in milk products. J. Dairy Sci. *42:* 945–960 (1958).

15 Kohn, R. R.: Principles of mammalian aging; in Kohn, (Prentice-Hall, Englewood Cliffs 1978).

16 Kuboki, Y.; Fujisawa, R.; Tsuzaki, M.; Liu, C. F.; Sasaki, S.: Presence of lysinoalanine and histidinoalanine in bovine dentin phosphoprotein. Calcif. Tissue. Int. *36:* 126–128 (1984).

17 Lepape, A.; Muh, J. P.; Bailey, A. J.: Characterization of N-glucosylated type 1 collagen in streptozotocin-induced diabetes. Biochem. J. *197:* 405–412 (1981).

18 Madia, A. M.; Rozovski, S. J.; Kagan, H. M.: Changes in lung lysyl oxidase activity in streptozotocin-diabetes and in starvation. Biochim biophys. Acta *585:* 481–487 (1979).

19 Mechanic, G. L.; Banes, A. J.; Henmi, M.; Yamauchi, M.: Possible collagen structural control of mineralization; in Butler, The chemistry and biology of mineralized tissues, pp. 98–102 (Ebsco Media, Alabama 1985).

20 Monnier, V. M.; Kohm, R. R.; Cerami, A.: Accelerated age-related browning of human collagen in diabetes mellitus. Proc. natn. Acad. Sci. USA *81:* 583–587 (1984).

21 Monnier, V. M.: The paradoxical effects of the Maillard reaction in vivo. Impaired maturation and accelerated aging of collagen. Proc. 3rd Int. Symp. on the Maillard Reaction, Tokyo 1985.

22 Moriguchi, T.; Fujimoto, D.: Age-related changes in the content of the collagen crosslink, pyridinoline. J. Biochem. *84:* 933–935 (1978).

23 Reynolds, T. M.: Chemistry of nonenzymic browning II. Adv. Food Res. *14:* 167–283 (1965).

24 Rigby, B. J.; Mitchell, T. W.; Robinson, M. S.: Oxygen participation in the in vivo and in vitro aging of collagen fibres. Biochem. biophys. Res. Commun. *79:* 400–405 (1977).

25 Sass, R. L.; Marsh, M. E.: N^τ-and N^π-histidinoalanine. Naturally occurring cross-linking amino acids in calcium-binding phophoproteins. Biochem. biophys. Res. Commun. *114:* 304–309 (1983).

26 Shikata, H.; Tsunoi, M.; Utsumi, N.; Hiramatsu, M.; Minami, N.; Fujimoto, D.: Effect of streptozotocin-induced diabetes mellitus on the content of crosslinked collagen in rat mandibular bone. Jap. J. oral Biol. *25:* 1164–1167 (1983).

27 Shikata, H.; Hiramatsu, M.; Masumizu, T.; Fujimoto, D.; Utsumi, N.: Age-related changes in the content of non-reducible crosslinks in rat mandibular bone. Archs oral Biol. *30:* 451–453 (1985).

28 Shikata, H.; Utsumi, N.; Hiramatsu, M.; Noguchi, M.; Fujimoto, D.: Effect of calcium deficiency on the content of non-reducible crosslinks in rat mandibular bone. Metabolism *35:* 206–208 (1986).

29 Siegel, R. C.; Fu, C. C.; Uto, N.; Horiuchi, K.; Fujimoto, D.: Collagen crosslinking. Lysyl oxidase dependent synthesis of pyridinoline. Confirmation that pyridinoline is derived from collagen. Biochem. biophys. Res. Commun. *108:* 1546–1550 (1982).

30 Sinex, F. M.: The role of collagen in aging; in Ramachandran, Treatise on collagen, vol. 2B, pp. 410–418 (Academic Press, New York 1968).

31 Sledge, C. V.: Formation and resorption of bone; in Kelley, Harris, Ruddy, Sledge, Textbook of rheumatology, pp. 277–293 (Saunders, Philadelphia 1981).

32 Tanzer, M. L.: Crosslinking of collagen; in Ramachandran, Reddi, Biochemistry of collagen, pp. 137–162 (Plenum Press, New York 1976).

33 Uchiyama, A.; Kushida, K.; Sumi, Y.; Deguchi, T.; Inoue, T.; Fujimoto, D.: Nonreducible crosslink and mineralization in bone. Biomed. Res. *4:* 257–260 (1983).

34 Yamauchi, M.; Banes, A. J.; Kuboki, Y.; Mechanic, G. L.: A comparative study of the distribution of stable crosslink, pyridinoline, in bone collagens from normal, osteoblastoma, and vitamin D-deficient chicks. Biochem. biophys. Res. Commun. *102:* 59–65 (1981).

H. Shikata, DDS, PhD, Jefferson Institute of Molecular Medicine, Department of Biochemistry, Jefferson Medical College of Thomas Jefferson University, Philadelphia, PA 19107 (USA)

Front. oral Physiol., vol. 6, pp. 96–110 (Karger, Basel 1987)

Protein Synthesis in Salivary Glands as Related to Aging

S. K. Kim

Research Service, VA Medical Center, and Department of Anatomy and Cell Biology, Medical School, Department of Oral Biology, School of Dentistry, The University of Michigan, Ann Arbor, Mich., USA

Introduction

The longevity of an organism is believed to be determined genetically by the number of cell divisions [19, 20] which are programmed in the constituent cells. However, many organs and tissues undergo a process of involution with age which leads to reductions in functions before they reach the maximum number of cell divisions [21]. Thus, the loss of cellular function may be considered to be the primary cause of aging at the organ or tissue level. An essential cellular function which has been shown to change with increasing age in various tissues and organs, including the salivary gland, is protein synthesis.

The alterations in the process of protein synthesis in salivary glands, or any other exocrine glands, would affect at least three different types of proteins; namely the secretory proteins, the structural proteins and the enzymes, some of which are involved in the synthesis of the above proteins. However, there is little information available regarding the age-related changes which are specific for the last two types of proteins in salivary glands. Therefore, the discussions presented in this chapter will deal exclusively with those changes which occur in relation to the synthesis of exportable, secretory proteins.

Overview of Changes in Protein Synthesis during Aging

The effects of aging on protein synthesis have been investigated in widely different tissues and organs of various organisms. The readers are referred to recent review articles by Richardson [65] and Reff [63] for detailed discussions on this subject. Only a brief summary of the general effects of aging on protein synthesis is presented here to provide the essential background for the discussions of protein synthesis in salivary glands.

The two prominent changes observed in various organs and tissues during aging are the decline in the rate of protein biosynthesis [63, 65] and the appearance of structurally altered proteins [63]. Both of these changes seem to occur in salivary glands in relation to aging. Consequently, these changes would affect cellular contents, as well as functional properties of glandular proteins.

The decline in rates of protein biosynthesis in relation to aging appears to be a change that is nearly universal in tissues of various eukaryotes [63, 65]. Studies dealing with rates of protein synthesis were largely performed using cell-free systems, cell suspensions or tissue slices obtained from the laboratory rat and mouse. Although there are studies demonstrating the increase in the rate of synthesis of certain proteins with age, such as the liver albumin [5, 14, 61], the majority of the work, based on the incorporation analysis of a labelled precursor into protein or acid-insoluble material, has shown that the rate of protein synthesis declines with age. This is especially true when the age of the animals is carefully selected and the changes in the size of the precursor pool are considered in calculating the rate of incorporation [65]. The age-related decline in the rate of protein synthesis has been reported in the liver [9, 12, 13, 24, 39, 40, 41, 46, 54, 64], muscles [7, 8, 69], brain [15, 26, 27, 55, 56], heart [16, 50], testis [43], kidney [5, 18], pancreas [32, 58] and salivary glands (see below).

This decline in the rate of protein synthesis during aging can be related to any number of changes at the level of transcription and translation. Those suggested changes during transcription involve the regulatory mechanism at the level of gene expression, but not the alterations (mutations) in the DNA itself [62]. Also, it has been suggested that changes in the binding between DNA and nucleoproteins [38, 70–72], or a shift in the nucleoproteins to a more basic arginine-rich protein [59, 72], cause reductions in rates of protein synthesis by repressing the gene activity.

The alterations implicated in the process of translation are mainly those which affect the rate of elongation of peptides, and include the decrease in the amino acylation of tRNA [47, 48, 75], the activity of one of the elongation factors [54], the initiation process due to the defects in a ribosomal subunit [12] and in the concentration of polysomes [69] or active ribosomes [40]. In addition, the decrease in the ribosome aggregation to messenger (mRNA) has been reported [41], and suggested to be related to the reductions in the availability of mRNA. Thus, it is uncertain what specific cellular changes cause the decline in the rate of protein synthesis during aging, or whether similar changes are responsible for this decline in different organs and tissues.

This statement of uncertainty also applies to the nature of cellular changes that cause alterations in protein molecules during aging. The protein molecules which are altered in physiological, chemical and biological properties occur in increasing frequency with age and accumulate in cells of aged organisms [1, 63]. These alterations can also occur due to changes at the level of transcription, translation or posttranslational processing. One possible mechanism by which altered proteins appear in cells is by the errors in the synthesis of these molecules, as was originally proposed by Orgel [60]. According to this theory, errors in the specificity of the proteins that are involved in the synthesis of other proteins produce faulty proteins, which, in turn, contribute in the increasing frequency of errors by a feedback type of mechanism. However, much of the existing evidence supports the view that the alterations in proteins probably occur post-translationally by modifications of the size, charge or conformation of correctly synthesized molecules [1, 63]. On the other hand, such modifications can also occur by aging of unaltered molecules as the molecules remain in older cells for a prolonged period due to reduced rates of synthesis and degradation or turnover.

Changes in the Rate of Protein Synthesis in Salivary Glands

Previous studies have reported that age-related reductions occur in the production, flow rate and protein content of the saliva. In addition, morphological changes which suggest reduced functions have been also reported to occur in salivary glands during aging. These changes will be discussed in detail in other chapters in this volume and will not be elaborated upon here. However, the alterations in the composition and secretion of saliva, as well as the structure of salivary glands, may reflect age-related changes in the process of protein synthesis.

Synthesis of Total Protein

As in other organs, one very prominent change which occur in salivary glands as a function of age is the progressive decline in rates of protein synthesis. This decline largely reflects the reduced rate of synthesis of secretory proteins. The studies of age-related changes in rates of protein biosynthesis in salivary glands were performed primarily by comparing rates of incorporation of labeled amino acids into acid-insoluble material (total protein) or into specific secretory proteins, using tissue slices or dispersed cells from laboratory rats. The maximum life span of these animals is about 4 years and the mortality rate at 24 months is about 50%.

Baum et al. [3], using dispersed cells of the submandibular gland, found that the rate of incorporation of radioactive amino acids into acid-insoluble material is significantly reduced in 24-month-old rats as compared to that in 4- to 6-month-old counterparts. Furthermore, the rate of intracellular processing of newly synthesized proteins is also reduced in the older group, especially that of a high molecular weight glycoprotein which appears to be the major secretory protein of the gland. It is not surprising to find parallel reductions in rates of synthesis and post-translational processing. Protein synthesis in salivary glands is one of several related cellular events in the secretory process, which includes processing, modification and packaging of newly synthesized proteins into granules and storage of these granules until their release upon stimulation. Thus, each event in the secretory process probably has a controlling effect on the other related events.

With the exception of the above mentioned study, the effects of aging on protein synthesis have been investigated mainly in the rat parotid gland. Kim and co-workers [30–32, 36, 37] have found that the rate of incorporation of radioactive leucine into acid-insoluble protein declines progressively with age in this gland. The rate of incorporation decreases gradually after 12 months reaching about 50% of the 2-month level at 30 months (fig. 1).

The reductions in rates of leucine incorporation in rat parotid glands represent actual decreases in rates of protein synthesis, and not the dilution of the specific activity of the amino acid due to age-related changes in the size of the precursor pool. There is no significant difference in the size of the intracellular free leucine pool in parotid glands of 2- and 24-month-old rats [36]. Furthermore, the specific activity of this pool in the older group is significantly higher than that in the younger counterpart [36]. However, the information regarding the precursor pool that serves as the direct source of amino acids for protein synthesis needs to be confirmed by measuring the specific activity of the transfer RNA-bound amino acid [65]. Unfortunately, the measurement of the specific activity of the amino acid bound to tRNA is hampered by the presence of a relatively high concentration of ribonucleases in parotid glands.

The age-related decline in the rate of protein synthesis in parotid glands does not reflect overall reductions in the metabolic or synthetic activity due to aging [30]. The ability of the gland slices to oxidize ^{14}C-glucose to $^{14}CO_2$, and to incorporate the label into total lipid does not change with age. On the other hand, the label incorporation into proteins

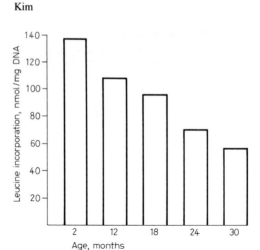

Fig. 1. Age-related changes in the rate of incorporation of leucine into acid-insoluble protein in rat parotid glands. The rate was calculated from the rate of incorporation of ³H-leucine during 1 h incubation.

decreases with age and parallels the decline in ³H-leucine incorporation. Further, the effect of aging on the rate of protein synthesis is not a reflection of the general deterioration affecting all aspects of the secretory function of the gland. Upon incubation of parotid lobules of 2- and 24-month-old rats in the presence of isoproterenol (IPR), these lobules release about the same proportions of tissue amylase at about the same rate [35]. The IPR-stimulated release is inhibited nearly completely by a β-blocking agent, propranolol, indicating that the release is mediated through β-adrenergic receptors. The above results indicate that the ability of the glandular cells to release secretory proteins remains unchanged with age and suggest that the reduction in the rate of protein synthesis in parotid glands is a specific age-related change.

Synthesis of Amylase and Other Secretory Proteins

As is expected, the age-related decline in the rate of protein synthesis in a secretory gland, such as the parotid gland, largely reflects the reduced rate of synthesis of exportable proteins [33, 34, 36]. The rate of synthesis of amylase, measured by incorporation of ³H-leucine into amylase after precipitation with glycogen [45], is significantly reduced in the glands of

Table I. Rate of amylase synthesis in stimulated and unstimulated parotid glands of young and old rats

Age months	Rats (number)	Rate of amylase synthesis ± SEM (number of experiments)
2	unstim. (4)	0.298 ± 0.012 (10)
	stim. (5)	0.298 ± 0.025 (7)
24	unstim. (5)	0.157 ± 0.014 (9)
	stim. (2)	0.271 ± 0.012 (4)

The data represent mean ± standard error of means. The rate of amylase synthesis was determined as the ratio of radioactivity incorporated into amylase to that into total protein of the gland. Amylase was precipitated with glycogen. From Kim [37] with the permission of Raven Press.

24-month-old rats as compared with that in 2-month-old rats [36]. In addition, the levels of radioactivity incorporated into amylase and other exportable secretory proteins are significantly lower in the older group when compared by radioactivity analysis of each band of proteins after electrophoretic separation in sodium dodecyl sulfate (SDS) containing gel [33, 34].

Protein Synthesis following Discharge of Stored Secretory Proteins

Previous studies have shown that the processes of synthesis and release of secretory proteins are interrelated in exocrine secretory cells, and that the rate of synthesis of these proteins increases greatly following the secretion of glandular contents [17, 42, 49, 67, 68]. The rat parotid gland can be induced to discharge nearly all stored secretory proteins by stimulating with a secretogogue, such as IPR [42]. Following this secretion, a burst of protein synthesis occurs and reaches its peak (2.5 times the prestimulation level) in about 6 h in parotid glands of young rats [42]. Thus, it is probable that the rate of protein synthesis in glands which are devoid of any stored proteins represents the true ability of cells to carry out this function. The reduced rate of synthesis in the glands of old rats may be related to a positive feedback type of inhibition [42] by the secretory proteins accumulating in cells due to the reduced level of secretion. In fact, the relatively high levels of amylase detected in glands of old rats [36, 37], despite significant reductions in the rate of protein synthesis, may be due to the accumulation of these proteins.

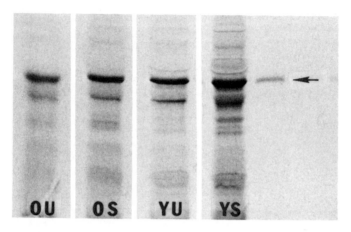

Fig. 2. Radioautograph of ^{35}S-methionine labeled proteins synthesized in a cell-free system, showing the differences in the translational activity of unfractionated RNA from unstimulated (U) and stimulated (S) parotid glands of 2-(Y) and 24-month-old (O) rats. The RNA from stimulated group was extracted 6 hs after stimulation with isoproterenol, at the time of maximum protein synthesis. Overall, the RNA from the younger group is much more efficient in directing translation. However, the translational activity of amylase mRNA in order rats increases to the level of the unstimulated young ones after stimulated secretion, as indicated by the intensity of the bands that comigrate with preamylase (arrow). The translation products were separated by electrophoresis in SDS containing polyacrylamide gel. Preamylase was synthesized in this system and immunoprecipitated using anti-amylase antibody.

Comparisons of rates of amylase synthesis in unstimulated and stimulated glands of young and old rats further support the possible regulation of secretory protein synthesis by a positive feedback type of mechanism [37]. The rate of amylase synthesis in unstimulated glands of 24-month-old rats, measured by determining the amount of radioactivity incorporated into this protein and expressing it as a percentage of that incorporated into total protein, is about one half of that in 2-month-old rats. However, the rate of amylase synthesis in parotid glands of the older rats increases to the level of the younger ones following the stimulated discharge of stored proteins (table I). These results suggest that the reduced rate of amylase synthesis in unstimulated glands of old rats is due to regulatory mechanisms in the cells which adjust the rate of synthesis of secretory proteins to balance with the reduced level of the secretory activity. If this is the case, then, it is also implied that the ability of secretory cells to synthesize secretory proteins remains unimpaired during aging.

Secretory Protein Synthesis and mRNA levels

One possible mechanism of the regulation of secretory protein synthesis involves mRNA specific for these proteins. The rate of synthesis of each protein appears to be proportional to the amount of the corresponding mRNA, and the level of mRNA stability clearly plays a leading role in the regulation of synthesis of most cellular proteins [44]. Thus, the changes in rates of protein synthesis in salivary glands during aging are likely to be related to the changes in the amount of mRNA available.

The analysis of unfractionated RNA from stimulated and unstimulated parotid glands of young and old rats by cell-free translation has shown that the increase in rate of amylase synthesis following stimulated secretion is accompanied by a similar increase in the messenger activity of amylase mRNA. The translational activity of amylase mRNA from stimulated glands of old rats is significantly greater than that from unstimulated glands and appears to be increased to the level of the RNA in the glands of young rats (fig. 2). Furthermore, cell-free translation analyses of unfractionated parotid RNA from 2-, 12- and 24-month-old rats have also indicated that the total messenger activity, as well as amylase mRNA activity, of the RNA from 24-month-old rats is considerably reduced as compared to that of the RNA from 2- and 12-month-old rats [37].

Whether or not the differences in the translational activity represent the actual differences in the amount of this RNA in parotid glands needs to be determined. Recent studies of liver mRNA using complementary DNA (cDNA) probes by Richardson et al. [66] have shown that the changes in the levels of synthesis of certain proteins during aging are accompanied by parallel changes in the amounts of mRNA species that code for these proteins. On the basis of these results, they have suggested that the changes in the levels of proteins during aging are regulated at the level of transcription.

Quantitative and Qualitative Changes in Secretory Proteins

Quantitative Changes

It is not unreasonable to expect a decrease in the level of secretory proteins in saliva and salivary glands in relation to the decline in the rate of protein synthesis during aging. In fact, it has been reported that reductions occur in the amylase content in saliva [11, 52, 53], as well as the secretion and rate of flow of saliva [6, 58] with increasing age in humans.

However, the information on the differences in salivary contents or output is variable [22] and not very valuable as an estimate of changes affecting protein synthesis in salivary glands. Such changes, even if proven to occur with age, may be related to the release mechanism of secretory proteins and not necessarily to the alterations in the reduced levels in glands.

On the other hand, the data obtained from the studies of secretory protein contents in salivary glands of laboratory animals are conflicting, and it is difficult to interpret correctly the differences in glandular contents of secretory proteins at any one moment because these levels represent the balance between synthesis and secretion or degradation [65]. In parotid glands of the rat, Kim [30, 31] has shown that glandular contents of amylase, determined by the assays of the enzyme activity, reduce with increasing age. Baum et al. [4] have confirmed this result using enzyme-linked immunosorbent assays and showed that the amylase contents decrease by about 50% between young (4–7 months) and old (24 months) ages. However, Kim et al. [36, 37] did not find any significant age-related changes when the glandular contents of amylase were assayed in rats which showed negative immunologic titers for the sialodacryoadenitis (SDA) virus. Since the rats used in the earlier study of Kim [30, 31] had positive SDA titers, the reduced levels of the enzyme in the old rats might have been related to the manifestation of this disease. The SDA virus is widely spread in many commercially available stocks of rats and is known to affect the structure and function of submandibular and parotid glands [25]. On the other hand, these discrepancies may represent actual variations among different strains of rats.

Qualitative Changes

Secretory proteins which are altered in their structure or function seem to appear with increasing frequency in saliva and salivary glands of aged humans and animals. It has been reported that acid DNase activity in parotid saliva collected from men and women over 50 years of age is significantly less than that of a younger group of individuals of 25–35 years of age [76]. However, the activity of neutral DNAse does not change significantly in these two age groups. A decrease in the sialic acid content has been reported to occur with increasing age in homogenates of submandibular glands in the rat [57]. In rat parotid glands, Chilla et al. [10] have detected 4 isoenzymes of amylase with different electrophoretic mobilities. Although the basic pattern of 4 isoenzymes was maintained, the activity of the 2 isoenzymes migrating faster towards the anode decreased significantly with increasing age.

α-Amylase is a glycoprotein consisting of a single chain of amino acids with a molecular weight of about 56,000 daltons [51]. The human parotid amylase consists of two families of isoenzymes which can be separated by disc-gel electrophoresis by differences in their molecular weights and carbohydrate contents [28, 29]. The A family consisting of 3 amylolytic bands contains covalently linked carbohydrates, while the B family of 2 isoenzymes and 2 forms of faster moving bands lack carbohydrates.

In addition to the basic pattern of these 6 isoenzymes, Arglebe et al. [2] have detected a group of isoamylases moving fast toward the anode in saliva collected from the parotid ducts of healthy men and women of varying ages. However, saliva from the older group (60–89 years of age) exhibits significantly more of these 'fast isoamylases' than that of the younger group (20–29 years of age). The increase in the amount of 'fast isoamylases' does not apparently affect the activity of amylase. Helfman and Price [23] reported that neither the specific activity nor the heat inactivation kinetics of α-amylase in the human saliva change with increasing age.

Therefore, it appears that molecules of isoamylases and some other secretory proteins altered in their structure and/or function, appear in human as well as rat glands. However, it is uncertain whether these altered isoamylases result from the age-related defects in mechanisms of the synthesis or post-translational processing of these molecules, or from aging of the basic isoamylases. Arglebe et al. [2] have suggested that the 'fast isoamylases' are derived from the basic isoenzymes by deamidation rather than by the synthesis of faulty proteins.

The isoenzymes of the parotid amylase can be transformed into more anionic forms by incubating at 37°C at alkaline pH [29], and this transformation seems to involve deamidation. Similarly, the incubation of pure pancreatric amylase at pH 9 and a temperature of 37°C results in deamidation of the asparagine and glutamine residues of the amylase molecule [51, 73, 74]. Furthermore, these fast moving (towards the anode), 'old isoamylases' can also be detected in the serum of patients with pancreatic pseudocysts, which are known to accumulate and store the pancreatic secretion rich in amylase [73, 74]. These results suggest that the increasing numbers of faster moving isoamylases appear in parotid saliva during aging as a consequence of prolonged storage of the enzyme in the gland rather than its faulty synthesis. However, there is no direct evidence that salivary gland cells of aged humans or animals do not synthesise faulty proteins. Therefore, the possibility cannot be ruled out that faulty secretory proteins appear because of an increasing frequency of errors in the synthesis or post-translational processing of these peptides during aging.

Concluding Remarks

The rate of protein synthesis declines with age in salivary glands as in many other organs and tissues. Furthermore, this decline largely reflects the reduced rate of synthesis of secretory proteins. Many possible changes at the level of transcription and translation can be the reasons for this decline in protein synthesis. It remains to be determined what specific changes cause the slowdown in protein synthesis in salivary glands. In addition, it is also possible that, in salivary glands, the decline is the result of a cellular regulatory mechanism of the secretory protein content, a positive feedback type of inhibition which compensates for the reduced level of secretory activity. The changes in the composition and secretion of saliva and the appearance of altered secretory proteins may be also related to deterioration in the process of protein synthesis during aging. However, no direct evidence linking the changes in protein synthesis to either quantitative or qualitative changes in secretory proteins has yet been produced.

References

1   Adelman, R. C.: Macromolecular metabolism during aging; in Finch, Hayflick, Handbook of the biology of aging, pp. 63–72 (van Nostrand Reinhold, New York 1977).

2   Arglebe, C.; Chilla, R.; Opaitz, M.: Age-dependent distribution of isoamylases in human parotid saliva. Clin. Otolaryyngol. *1:* 249–256 (1976).

3   Baum, B. J.; Kuyatt, B. L.; Humphreys, S.: Protein production and processing in young adult and aged rat submandibular gland cells in vitro. Mech. Age. Dev. *23:* 123–136 (1983).

4   Baum, B. J.; Levine, R. L.; Kuyatt, B. L.; Sogin, D. B.: Rat parotid gland amylase: evidence for alterations in an exocrine protein with increasing age. Mech. Age. Dev. *19:* 27–35 (1982).

5   Beauchene, R. E.; Roeder, L. M.; Barrows, C. H.: The interrelationship of age, tissue protein synthesis, and proteinuria. J. Geront. *25:* 359–363 (1970).

6   Bertram, U.: Xerostomia: clinical aspects, pathology and pathogenesis. Acta odont. scand. *25:* suppl. 49, pp. 1–126 (1967).

7   Breuer, C. B.; Florini, J. R.: Amino acid incorporation into protein by cell-free systems from rat skeletal muscle. IV. Effects of animal age, androgens, and anabolic agents on activity of muscle ribosomes. Biochemistry *4:* 1544–1550 (1965).

8   Britton, G. W.; Sherman, F. G.: Altered regulation of protein synthesis during aging as determined by in vitro ribosomal assays. Exp. Gerontol. *10:* 67–77 (1975).

9   Buetow, D. E.; Gandhi, P. S.: Decreased protein synthesis by microsomes isolated from senescent rat liver. Exp. Gerontol. *8:* 243–249 (1973).

10   Chilla, R.; Arglebe, C.; Domagk, G. F.: Age-dependent changes in the alpha-isoamylase pattern of human and rat parotid glands. Oto-Rhino-Laryngol. *36:* 373–382 (1974).

11   Chilla, R.; Niemann, H.; Arglebe, C.; Domagk, G. F.: Age-dependent changes in the alpha-isoamylase pattern of human and rat parotid glands. Oto-Rhino-Laryngol. *36:* 372–382 (1974).

12   Comolli, R.: Deficiency in accessory protein of native 40S ribosomal subunits in the liver of aging rats. Exp. Gerontol. *10:* 31–36 (1975).

13   Comolli, R.; Delpiano, C.; Shubert, A. C.: Dependency on the source of supernatant factors for optimal ^{14}C-polyphenylalanine synthesis by high salt treated liver ribosomal subunits in rats of different ages. Exp. Gerontol. *11:* 5–10 (1976).

14   Coniglio, J. J.; Liu, D. S. H.; Richardson, A.: A comparison of protein synthesis by liver parenchymal cells isolated from Fischer F344 rats of various ages. Mech. Age. Dev. *11:* 77–90 (1979).

15   Ekstrom, R.; Liu, D. S. H.; Richardson, A.: Changes in brain protein synthesis during the life span of male Fischer rats. Gerontology *26:* 121–128 (1980).

16   Geary, S.; Florini, J. R.: Effect of age on rate of protein synthesis in isolated perfused mouse hearts. J. Geront. *27:* 325–332 (1972).

17   Grand, R. J.; Gross, P. R.: Independent stimulation of secretion and protein synthesis in rat parotid gland. J. biol. Chem. *244:* 5608–5615 (1969).

18   Hardwick, J.; Heish, W. H.; Liu, D. S. H.; Richardson, A.: Cell-free protein synthesis by rat kidney: the effect of age on kidney protein synthesis. Biochem. biophys. Acta *652:* 204–217 (1981).

19   Hayflick, L.; Moorhead, P. S.: The serial cultivation of human diploid cell strains. Exp. Cell Res. *25:* 585–621 (1961).

20   Hayflick, L.: The limited in vitro life time of human diploid cell strains. Exp. Cell Res. *37:* 614–636 (1965).

21   Hayflick, L.: Cell aging; in Cherkin et al., Physiology and cell biology of aging. Aging, vol. 8, pp. 3–19 (Raven Press, New York 1979).

22   Heft, M. W.; Baum, B. J.: Unstimulated and stimulated parotid salivary flow rate in individuals of different ages. J. dent. Res. *63:* 1182–1185 (1984).

23   Helfman, P. M.; Price, P. A.: Human parotid α-amylase – a test of the error theory of aging. Exp. Gerontol. *9:* 204–214 (1974).

24   Hrachovec, J. P.: Age changes in amino acid incorporation by rat liver microsomes. Gerontologia *15:* 52–63 (1969).

25   Jonas, A. M.; Craft, J.; Black, C. L.; Bhatt, P. N.; Hilding, D.: Sialodacryoadenitis in the rat. A light and electron microscopic study. Archs Path. *88:* 613–622 (1969).

26   Johnson, T. C.: Cell-free protein synthesis by mouse brain during early development. J. Neurochem. *15:* 1189–1194 (1968).

27   Johnson, T. C.; Belytschko, G.: Alteration in microsomal protein synthesis during early development of mouse brain. Proc. natn. Acad. Sci. USA *62:* 844–851 (1969).

28   Kauffman, D. L.; Zager, N. I.; Cohen, E.; Keller, P. J.: The isozymes of human parotid amylase. Archs Biochem. Biophys. *137:* 325–339 (1970).

29   Keller, P. J.; Kauffman, D. L.; Allan, B. J.; Williams, B. L.: Further studies on the structural differences between the isozymes of human parotid α-amylase. Biochemistry *10:* 4867–4874 (1971).

30   Kim, S. K.; Weinhold, P. A.; Han, S. S.; Wagner, D. J.: Age-related decline in protein synthesis in the rat parotid gland. Exp. Gerontol. *15:* 71–85 (1980).

31   Kim, S. K.: Age-related changes of amylase and protein synthesis in the rat parotid gland. J. dent. Res. *60:* 738–749 (1981).

32   Kim, S. K.; Weinhold, P. A.; Calkins, D. W.; Hartog, V. W.: Comparative studies of the age-related changes in protein synthesis in the rat pancreas and parotid gland. Exp. Gerontol. *16:* 91–100 (1981).

33   Kim, S. K.; Calkins, D. W.; Weinhold, P. A.; Han, S. S.: The changes in the synthesis of exportable and nonexportable proteins in parotid glands during aging. Mech. Age. Dev. *18:* 239–250 (1982).

34   Kim, S. K.; Calkins, D. W.; Secretory protein synthesis in parotid glands of young and old rats. Archs oral Biol. *28:* 1–4 (1983).

35   Kim, S. K.; Calkins, D. W.; Weinhold, P. A.: Secretion of α-amylase from parotid lobules of young and old rats. Exp. Gerontol. *17:* 387–397 (1983).

36   Kim, S. K.: The synthesis of α-amylase in parotid glands of young and old rats. Mech. Age. Dev. *31:* 257–266 (1985).

37   Kim, S. K.: The synthesis of secretory proteins in parotid glands of young and old rats; in Sohal et al., Molecular biology of aging: gene stability and gene expression, pp. 291–306 (Raven Press, New York 1985).

38   Kurtz, D. K.; Sinex, F. M.: Age-related differences in the association of brain DNA and nuclear protein. Biochim. biophys. Acta *145:* 840–842 (1967).

39   Kurtz, D. I.: The effect of ageing on in vitro fidelity of translation in mouse liver. Biochim. biophys. Acta *407:* 479–484 (1975).

40   Kurtz, D. I.: A decrease in the number of active mouse liver ribosomes during aging. Exp. Gerontol. *13:* 397–402 (1978).

41   Layman, D. K.; Ricca, G. A.; Richardson, A.: The effect of age on protein synthesis and ribosome aggregation to messenger RNA in rat liver. Archs Biochem. Biophys. *173:* 246–254 (1976).

42   Lillie, J. H.; Han, S. S.: Secretory protein synthesis in the stimulated rat parotid gland. J. Cell Biol. *59:* 708–721 (1973).

43   Liu, D. S. H.; Ekstrom, R.; Spicer, J. W.; Richardson, A.: Age-related changes in protein, RNA and DNA content and protein synthesis in rat testes. Exp. Gerontol. *13:* 197–205 (1978).

44   Lodish, H. F.: Translational control of protein synthesis. A. Rev. Biochem. *45:* 39–72 (1976).

45   Loyter, A.; Schramm, M.: The glycogen-amylase complex as a means of obtaining highly purified α-amylases. Biochim. biophys. Acta *65:* 201–206 (1962).

46   Mainwaring, W. I. P.: The effect of age on protein synthesis in mouse liver. Biochem. J. *113:* 869–878 (1969).

47   Mariotti, D.; Ruscitto, R.: Age-related changes of accuracy and efficiency of protein synthesis machinery in rat. Biochim. biophys. acta *475:* 96–102 (1977).

48   Mays, L. L.; Lawrence, A. E.; Ho, R. W.; Ackley, S.: Age-related changes in function of transfer ribonucleic acid of rat liver. Fed. Proc. *38:* 1984–1988 (1979).

49   McPherson, M. A.; Hales, C. N.: Control of amylase biosynthesis and release in the parotid gland of the rat. Biochem. J. *176:* 855–863 (1978).

50   Meerson, F. Z.; Javich, M. P.; Lerman, M. I.: Decrease in the rate of RNA and protein synthesis and degradation in the myocardium under long-term compensatory hyperfunction and on aging. J. mol. cell. Cardiol. *10:* 145 (1978).

51   Merritt, A. D.; Karn, R. C.: The human α-amylases; in Harris, Hirschhorn, Advances in human genetics, pp. 135–235 (Plenum Press, New York 1982).

52   Meyer, J.; Necheles, H.: Studies in old age. IV. The clinical significance of salivary, gastric and pancreatic secretion in the aged. J. Am. med. Ass. *115:* 2050–2053 (1940).

53   Meyer, J.; Golden, J. S.; Steiner, N.; Necheles, H.: The ptyalin content of human saliva in old age. Am. J. Physiol. *119:* 600–602 (1937).

54   Moldave, K.; Harris, J.; Sabo, W.; Sadnik, I.: Protein synthesis and aging: studies with cell-free mammalian systems. Fed. Proc. *38:* 1979–1983 (1979).

55   Murthy, M. R. V.; Rappoport, D. A.: Biochemistry of the developing rat brain. V.

Cell-free incorporation of L-[I-^{14}C]-leucine into microsomal protein. Biochim. biophys. Acta 95: 121–131 (1965).

56 Murthy, M. R. V.: Protein synthesis in growing rat tissues. II. Polyribosome concentration of brain and liver as a function of age. Biochim. biophys. Acta 119: 599–613 (1966).

57 Mysliwski, A.; Zurawska-Czupa, B.: Concentration of sialic acids in submandibular glands of young and old rats treated with isoproterenol. Exp. Gerontol. 11: 149–152 (1976).

58 Necheles, H.; Plotke F.; Meyer, J.: Studies on old age. V. Active pancreatic secretion in the aged. Am. J. dig. Dis. 9: 157–159 (1942).

59 O'Meara, A. R.; Herrmann, R. L.: A modified mouse liver chromatin preparation dsplaying age-related differences in salt dissociation and template ability. Biochim. biophys. Acta 269: 419–427 (1972).

60 Orgel, L. E.: The maintenance of the accuracy of protein synthesis and its relevance to ageing. Proc. natn. Acad. Sci. USA 49: 517–521 (1963).

61 Ove, P.; Obenrader, M.; Lansing, A.: Synthesis and degradation of liver proteins in young and old rats. Biochim. biophys. Acta 277: 211–221 (1972).

62 Pyhtila, M. J.; Sherman, F. G.: Age-associated studies on thermal stability and template effectiveness of DNA and nucleoproteins from beef thymus. Biochem. biophys. Res. Commun. 31: 340–344 (1968).

63 Reff, M. E.: RNA and protein metabolism; in Finch, Schneider, Handbook of the biology of aging; 2nd ed., pp. 225–254 (van Nostrand Reinhold, 1985).

64 Ricca, G. A.; Liu, D. S. H.; Coniglio, J. J.; Richardson, A.: Rate of protein synthesis by hepatocytes isolated from rats of various stages. J. cell. Physiol. 97: 137–146 (1978).

65 Richardson, A.: The relationship between aging and protein synthesis; in Florini, Handbook of biochemistry in aging, pp. 79–101 (1981).

66 Richardson, A.; Rutherford, M. S.; Birchenall-Sparks, M. C.; Roberts, M. S.; Wu, W. T.; Cheung, H. T.: Levels of specific messenger RNA species as a function of age; in Sohal et al., Molecular biology of aging: gene stability and gene expression, pp. 229–241 (Raven Press, New York 1985).

67 Rosenfeld, M. G.; Abrass, I. B.; Chang, B.: Hormonal stimulation of alpha-amylase synthesis in porcine pancreatic minces. Endocrinology 99: 611–618 (1976).

68 Sreebny, L. M.; Johnson, D. A.; Robinovitch, M. R.: Functional regulation of protein synthesis in the rat parotid gland. J. biol. Chem. 246: 3879–3884 (1971).

69 Srivastava, U.: Polyribosome concentration of mouse skeletal muscle as a function of age. Archs Biochem. Biophys. 130: 129–139 (1969).

70 von Hahn, H. P.: Stabilization of DNA structure by histones against thermal denaturation. Experentia 21: 90–91 (1965).

71 von Hahn, J. P.; Fritz, E.: Age-related alterations in the structure of DNA. 3. Thermal stability of rat liver DNA related to age, histone content and ionic strength. Gerontologia 12: 237–250 (1966).

72 von Hahn, H. P.; Miller, J.; Eichhorn, G. L.: Age-related alterations in the structure of nucleoprotein. IV. Changes in the composition of whole histone from rat liver. Gerontologia 15: 293–301 (1969).

73 Warshaw, A. L.; Lee, K.–H.: Aging changes of pancreatic isoamylases and the appearance of 'old amylase' in the serum of patients with pancreatic pseudocysts. Gastroenterology 79: 1246–1251 (1980).

74 Weaver, D. W.; Bouwman, D. L.; Walt, A. J.: Aged amylase. A valuable test for detecting and tracking pancreatic pseudocysts. Archs. Surg., Chicago 117: 707–711 (1982).

75 Wust, C. J.; Rosen, L.: Aminoacylation and methylation of tRNA as a function of age in the rat. Exp. Gerontol. *7:* 331–343 (1972).
76 Yaegaki, K.; Sakata, T.; Ogura, R.; Kameyama, T.; Sujaku, C.: Influence of aging on DNase activity in human parotid saliva. J. Dent. Res. *61:* 1222–1224 (1982).

S. K. Kim, PhD, Research Service, VA Medical Center, and Department of Anatomy and Cell Biology, Medical School, Department of Oral Biology, School of Dentistry, The University of Michigan, Ann Arbor, MI 48105 (USA)

Front. oral Physiol., vol. 6, pp. 111–125 (Karger, Basel 1987)

Collagen Changes in Dental Pulp

C. J. Nielsen

'This streptococcus business is getting me addlepated.
Will you please tell me whether you think the streptococcus
is really a result or a cause.'

Author unknown, ca. 1932

Introduction

Like the addlepated author above, anyone who has tried to stay abreast of recent advances in the field of connective tissue changes within the dental pulp may face a fair amount of addlepation of his own. Freshmen dental students of a generation ago could rest easily in the knowledge that the dental pulp did indeed fibrose with age. However, as improvements in tools and techniques have advanced, so has the body of information with regard to age changes in pulpal connective tissue, particularly pulpal collagen. This is, of course, as one would expect realizing the rapid advancement in knowledge over the same time period regarding the protein's chemical characterization and biosynthesis. Nevertheless, the opportunity for confusion exists as the literature on the subject has a fair amount of inconsistency. Does the pulp 'contain very small amounts of collagen' [35] or a 'relatively large amount of collagen' [14]? Are we to believe that 'the dental pulp is unlike most connective tissue in its composition' [36] or that 'pulpal connective tissue is similar in composition, organization, and histochemical reactivity to other connective tissue' [61]? In any case no longer is it enough to know that the pulp becomes increasingly fibrous with age. Now the serious pulp biologist wants to know if particular areas are more susceptible to fibrosis, if particular collagen types are associated with dental developmental patterns, or if certain pathophysiologic states can be explained in terms of changes in the connective tissue matrix. Over the past few years the whole area of 'ground substance' and its relation to the protein is only beginning to be understood. The facts being discovered today are not entirely consistent with the beliefs of a generation ago. Does the pulp proper truly fibrose with age? Is pulp connective tissue as unique a tissue as some would have us believe or is it basically similar to other connective tissue throughout the body? The intent of this chapter is to bring together recent developments in pulp collagen research and where possible, try to fit new ideas in with earlier held beliefs and observations. In certain instances, more questions than answers may arise and we will have to look to the future before we can expect further explanations.

Light Microscopy

Earliest descriptive accounts of changes in pulp collagen and its relation to surrounding connective tissue involved the use of the light microscope. There was almost universal agreement that with age pulp tissue in general showed a decrease in cellularity with an increase in collagen fiber content. As more research was published a distinction became apparent between coronal and radicular pulp collagen concentration and morphology. In 1962, Stanley and Ranney [49] described two variations of collagen fiber types: one, 'diffuse' collagen, was a lacey network with no definitive orientation and another, 'bundle' collagen, whose coarse fibers ran parallel to nerves or independently. Their work also found more collagen fibers in anterior teeth in general and less collagen in coronal pulp tissue than radicular pulp. The amount of coronal pulp collagen did not increase after age 20 and the authors were surprised to see how little collagen was found in the coronal pulps of older (over 50 years of age) intact posterior teeth. 'Diffuse' collagen of the root seemed to decrease between the ages of 10 and 49 years. The authors felt that any changes in collagen were probably not due to aging but instead were a reaction to previous irritation and/or stimulation of the pulp.

Bhussry [7] found an increase in the amount of collagen in the subodontoblastic layer of pulps of old teeth. In the center of the pulp chamber were noted scattered areas of collagen bundle formation while younger teeth had diffuse distribution of varying amounts of collagen. Reticular fibers were seen to increase uniformly in all areas of the pulp. The most significant histological changes occurred during development and maturation and very little during aging.

The reticular nature of young coronal pulp was also emphasized by Bernick and Nedelman [5] who found the zone of Weil to be free of any argyrophilic fiber concentration. The only collagen bundles to be seen were adventitial and neural sheaths. With age and calcification of vessels and nerves, there was a decrease in such elements leaving only their connective tissue sheaths giving the coronal pulp an increasingly fibrotic appearance. The stroma of the pulp nevertheless consisted of fine collagenous fibers regardless of age. (Provenza [41] argued against pulp vessels having a true adventitial sheath. He suggested that any fibrous outer coat of a vessel in the pulp consisted of the very fine reticulin-like stroma through which the vessel passed. While his argument would not be accepted by many pulp biologists of today, it certainly lent credence to another misconception that due to lack of a strong vessel wall, increased intrapulpal pressure arising from inflammation could strangulate the pulp. Of course the work of Van Hassel [59] has largely discredited such an idea.)

Zerlotti [61] in a histochemical analysis of the pulp suggested an increase in the amount of collagen by referring to aged pulps as having an extracellular matrix formed mostly of collagenous bundles. Collagen fibers replaced to a large extent the argyrophilic fibers and ground substance. The author suggested that the absence of argyrophilia with age could be related to the protein's maturation as the fibers lost part of their carbohydrate fraction and became more cross-linked. This suggestion is supported by the more recent report of decreasing hydroxylysyl glycoside (collagen associated carbohydrate) levels in the maturing bovine pulp [40].

In summary, fibrosis of the pulp, in particular the radicular pulp, appears to be fact when viewed under the light microscope. The etiology of this fibrosis remains in question however. Diminishing pulpal volume could certainly contribute to the apparent increase. Does the pulp continue to produce collagen at a constant rate throughout its life and thereby account for the fibrosis? As the reader will see shortly, the tissue not only diminishes its rate of synthesis, but it also successfully diminishes its total collagen content, if not its concentration.

Electron Microscopy

Beginning in the early 1960s the electron microscope had begun adding to our knowledge of the dental pulp in general and pulp collagen synthesis and morphology specifically. The odontoblast in particular proved to be a unique and invaluable aid in studying ultrastructural relationships between the cell's collagen synthesis and the protein's final utilization in hard tissue deposition. The work of many authors has elaborated on the ultrastructure of dental fibroblasts and collagen fibers in both developing and mature human and animal pulp. The reader is referred to the works of others [1, 2, 16] for further detail.

In 1961, Avery and Han [3] investigated young hamster molar pulps and found what they believed to be young collagen fibers in contact with fibroblast cell membranes. Intracytoplasmic filaments near the surface of these cells were thought to probably play a role in fibrogenesis. Han and Avery [18] in 1965 using guinea pig incisors found collagen fibrils ranging in diameter from 400 to 700 Å in addition to a fine fibril of 100–200 Å. Two distinct collagen fibers were noted by Harris and Griffin [20]; one of 700 A diameter found in younger pulps, the other of 778 Å diameter found in mature pulps.

The question arises in many of these studies whether the smaller fibrils in certain circumstances aggregate to form the larger fibers with the passage of time. Certain factors which might modulate such aggregation are proximity to cells [3, 18], electrical and physical forces acting within the ground substance [18], or the ground substance itself [16, 17]. While fibril aggregation has yet to be conclusively proven in the pulp, the possibility that such does occur correlates well with the decrease in reticular fibers noted by some authors [49, 61] using light microscopy and the decrease in the protein's solubility to be discussed shortly.

Electron microscopy also indicated that as the pulp ages the fibroblast cell population of a given tooth undergoes maturation. Harris and Griffin [20] differentiated between two types of fibroblasts, young and mature. The former cells had mitochondria of diameter 4,645 Å with a predominence of cisternal vesicles. Their function appeared to be the synthesis of beaded microfibrils. The mature cells tended to possess more organelles, aggregations of smooth-walled vesicles at the plasma membrane, and increasing numbers of cytoplasmic ribosomes. They appeared to be in the process of elaborating soluble collagen. Han et al. [19] also distinguished between pulpal fibroblasts using the continuously growing guinea pig incisor. Their study noted three stages: early differentiation, maturation and functioning, and finally, regression.

In an investigation of human teeth [9] from patients of ages 12–60 a similar distinction is made between young and old fibroblasts. Young cells were characterized by numerous fine intracytoplasmic fibrils and organelles including rough endoplasmic reticulum, Golgi apparatus, and mitochondria. Older pulps had cells with few organelles and a lack of intracytoplasmic fibrils. Breyan and Schilder [8] in a comparison of 'young' pulps of the continuously growing rat incisor with 'mature' pulp of a 19-year-old human found the former tissue to have very active fibroblasts engaged in the synthesis of collagen precursors. The human fibroblast displayed a more passive role as the extracellular segregation of collagen molecules was completed.

From these ultrastructural studies it became apparent that the collagen produced by the pulpal fibroblast might well aggregate into larger fibers with time. The increasingly fibrotic nature of the radicular pulp seen under the light microscope would support this view. Furthermore, pulpal fibroblasts appeared to undergo a maturation process of their own, ultimately resulting in a decrease of their own number and thereby accounting for the decrease in total cell population noted by numerous authors [24, 54]. It is no wonder that the ability of the pulp to produce collagen diminishes with age [34, 39, 57]. Yet neither light nor electron microscopy could answer the question of whether or not increased fiber formation represented a relative or absolute increase in collagen content. The method by which the query would be answered lay in more direct biochemical assay procedures.

Pulp Collagen Content

Attempts to measure absolute amounts of pulpal collagen and collagen concentration have been relatively few. The results achieved to date are difficult to apply to the human situation because different animal models were used and results reported in differing units. Uitto and Antila [56] investigated rabbit molar and incisor pulp and found collagen to be 0.69 and 0.52% of wet weight, respectively. The ratio of collagen to total protein was 12.0 and 10.3%. Orlowski [35] stated that collagen was 12.7% of dry weight in porcine pulp and 16.8% in bovine pulp. He subsequently found the rat incisor to have 3.3–4.7% collagen and the molar to have 7.0% collagen on a dry weight basis [36, 37]. In an investigation of human pulp specimens it was determined that collagen accounted for 'about 25% of the dry mass' and 'about 3.5% of the wet weight' [58].

None of these investigations compared collagen concentration over a period of time and studies doing so are even fewer. Using bovine pulp taken from teeth over the entire age range of the animal Hayakawa et al. [22] showed that in terms of dry weight collagen concentration does increase from 9 to 25%. Total collagen per pulp, however, ultimately diminished from around 30 mg/pulp at the stage of half-root development to approximately 4 mg/pulp at the stage of attrition. Leichner and Kalnitsky [29], again using bovine pulp, found a similar increase in collagen concentration from 15.2% of dry weight in embryonic tissue to 23% of dry weight in mature tissue.

Uitto and Ranta [57] in a comparison of human bicuspids with roots either incompletely or completely formed found that the concentration of collagen increased with age both in terms of wet weight (1.44–2.08%) and total protein (30.0–37.1%). (As in many studies this one in fact looked at more than one variable. Attempting to measure wet weights of human pulp tissue is difficult at best. Assessing changes in the collagen/

protein ratio can also be open to interpretation. Any increase can be a result of two occurrences. The pulp may be producing more collagen in relation to total protein as the study suggests or the tissue may be producing less total protein with time and thereby giving the appearance of an increase in the collagen/protein ratio.) Like Hayakawa's et al. [22] study this one also reports a reduction (by 48%) in total collagen per pulp between the stages of early and complete root development. Finally, in an investigation of human third molars, Nielsen et al. [34] found no change in coronal pulp collagen concentration in terms of protein over the ages of 15–40 years.

There seems to be little doubt that the rate of collagen synthesis decreases as the pulp ages. Three investigations, one by Uitto and Ranta [57] measuring proline hydroxylase activity in human pulp, one by Nielsen et al. [34] measuring changes in reducible collagen cross-link concentrations in human pulp, and one by Patten et al. [39] studying the incorporation of ^{3}H-proline into bovine pulp, all show that with age the tissue produces increasingly less collagen.

The general consensus appears to be that the increased fibrosis as evaluated with the light microscope does indeed occur with time. This is reflected in an increased concentration of the protein albeit the total amount of collagen per pulp decreases. While diminishing pulpal volume cannot be ruled out as a cause of increased concentration, as we will see shortly, the protein's diminishing solubility supports the idea of increasing aggregation of fibrils due to increasing intermolecular bond formation.

Pulp Collagen Solubility

In contrast to the majority of proteins the biologic half-life of collagen is very long and as a result it is possible to study time-dependent changes in its physical properties. Shortly after secretion from the cell, collagen molecules aggregate to form fibrils and fiber bundles as part of the connective tissue matrix. Maturation of the protein with time involves formation of covalent cross-links between molecules which increase its stability to external influences such as extraction procedures.

Numerous studies have reported pulp collagen's decreasing solubility. Shuttleworth et al. [47], using a pepsin digestion method, analyzed the protein's solubility from two stages of development of bovine pulp, papilla and mature pulp. 80% of the total collagen could be solubilized from the embryonic tissue of the papilla compared to only 65% of the mature pulp. In a histochemical study of human teeth at different ages Zerlotti [61] found the soluble fraction of the protein decreased by a factor of ten between a one-year-old and older age groups. An increase in the resistance to proteolytic enzymes was also noted. These decreases in solubility, however, may be in part related to the type of tooth one studies. Shuttleworth et al. [48] showed that while bovine molar pulp collagen becomes increasingly resistant to solubilization, rabbit incisor collagen fails to show any decrease. Aside from the obvious species difference, the authors attribute the finding to the fact that the incisor is a continuously growing organ with a much higher rate of collagen synthesis [38] than the molar. The lower solubility of the molar collagen might be due to the greater incorporation of soluble collagen into the insoluble network with time as suggested by Uitto and Antilla [56] who speculated that molar collagen may become cross-linked faster than that of the incisor. In the continuously erupting incisor the greater amount of soluble collagen could be a result of a higher proportion of newly synthesized protein. In either case the evidence points to increasing intermolecular cross-links decreasing the protein's solubility as the pulp ages.

The major stabilizing cross-links between collagen molecules result from Schiff base condensations between one of two aldehydic residues, allysine or hydroxyallysine, formed by the action of the connective tissue enzyme, lysyl oxidase, and either a lysyl or hydroxylysyl residue. Depending on which two of the four residues combine, one of three aldimines can be created: dehydrolysinonorleucine, dehydrohydroxylysinonorleucine, or dehydrodihydroxylysinonorleucine. These in turn after hydrolysis and reduction in a test tube give rise to the reduced forms of lysinonorleucine (LNL), hydroxylysinonorleucine (HLNL), and dihydroxylysinonorleucine (DHLNL). In general LNL is a minor component of any tissue while DHLNL is most prominent in hard tissue such as bone or dentin.

In the past few years several investigations of pulpal collagen cross-link patterns have emerged. In 1975, Takagi et al. [52], studying bovine pulp from animals 1–4 years of age, found the ratio of DHLNL to HLNL to increase from 0.82 at age one to 1.33 at age four. Takagi [51], again using bovine pulp, reported the ratio to be 0.37 (age?) while Kuboki et al. [27] gave a ratio of 0.49 for 4-year-old bovine pulp. The close similarity of this ratio to that of skin (0.66) compared to that found in bone or dentine (2.3 and 6.0, respectively) led Kuboki et al. [27] to speculate whether pulpal collagen was not more similar to the collagen found in other soft tissues.

In an investigation of human third molar coronal pulps ranging in patient age from 15 to 40 years. Nielsen et al. [34] found DHLNL to be the major cross-link in the pulp throughout the span of the study. Using the premise of Robins et al. [43], that the presence of reducible cross-links is indicative of collagen synthesis, they concluded based on diminishing levels of DHLNL that the rate of the synthesis of the protein decreases within coronal pulp as the tissue matures.

The presence of DHLNL in any tissue will have a bearing on that tissue's solubility [42]. Because of its ability to undergo an Amadori rearrangement to the more stable keto form this cross-link renders the fibers more stable than does either HLNL or LNL. If the collagen of pulp tissue is less soluble than collagens of other tissues as some would suggest [50, 58] this might be attributable in part to the higher percentage of DHLNL cross-links within the pulp.

The preceding discussion is of interest when applied to a theoretical explanation of a hitherto incompletely explained clinical observation. Any dentist providing a large amount of endodontic therapy for his patients has more than likely encountered the situation of initiating endodontic treatment on a badly carious tooth (usually a molar in a young adult in the author's practice) with what appears to be radiographic evidence of periapical involvement. On occasion, to the practitioner's surprise, upon opening the pulp chamber he finds a reasonably intact pulp when from the radiograph he anticipated finding a much less viable looking tissue. (The author believes it a fair assertion to state that in the presence of radiographic periapical pathology, the contents of the chamber and canal are usually necrotic or characterized by total chronic pulpitis. Certainly the near reverse is true, that if the chamber and canal contents are necrotic or if total pulpitis exists, then the apical area is always involved at least histologically [45].)

Several references [25, 30, 31, 33] in the literature report evidence of vital tissue existing in the presence of periapical pathology. Jordan et al. [25] and Moore [33] successfully maintained pulp vitality even with preoperative conditions of periapical radiolucency. Bender et al. [4], in a histological study of such teeth, found inflammation in the coronal portion subjacent to caries but uninflamed tissue in the radicular portion of the pulp. The periapical region was described as having an infiltrate of chronic inflammatory cells (fig. 1). In an attempt to explain the observation of two sites of inflammation arising from a single source and separated by seemingly normal tissue, Seltzer et al. [46] speculated that the fibrous collagen bundles of radicular pulp were responsible for limiting progression of the inflammatory infiltrate into the root portion of the tissue. Nevertheless, some chronic inflammatory cells were still found in the periapical area. Langeland et al. [28] attributed the appearance of periapical inflammation in the presence of relatively unaltered radicular pulp tissue to the presence of lymph vessels which carried tissue dis-

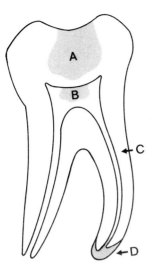

Fig. 1. In a young tooth caries (A) may promote an inflammatory response both in the pulp chamber (B) and the periapical area (D) and yet radicular pulp (C) remains uninflamed. See text for further discussion.

integration products and bacterial toxins past the radicular portion into the periapical area.

Both of these concepts, the fibrous nature of the radicular pulp and lymphatic drainage to the periapical area, may account for what is seen histologically and clinically. The author however would like to suggest another possible contributing factor which concerns the nature of the tissues involved. It might be argued that the periapical area in young individuals is inherently more susceptible to inflammatory changes than is radicular pulp because of its more recent development. Different authorities place final morphogenic root closure of a first molar anywhere between 9 and 12 years of age [13, 25]. What exactly is the nature of the tissue directly apical to the last remnant of epithial diaphragm (Hertwig's root sheath)? Because the apical foramen has closed are we to assume the soft tissue has reached full maturity? Would this tissue not be the last remnants of dental papilla prior to the inductive effect of the root sheath? As such it is a more immature tissue than the pulp as evidenced by the papilla being more susceptible to extraction procedures [47]. With cementum having been laid down only recently the completed periodontal ligament has just begun to form in the area as fibers become continuous between cementum and bone.

The percentage of DHLNL to HLNL in the ligament is reported to be less than in pulp in at least one study [27]. If DHLNL does provide for a more stable collagen fiber as already discussed, the lower DHLNL/ HLNL ratio in the periodontal ligament might suggest that this tissue is more soluble than pulp. Furthermore, the apical area is one of rapid tooth formation and as such must be involved in rapid collagen synthesis [57]. High levels of synthesis of the protein are associated with high levels of turnover [36]. In an area of high turnover, the ability of collagen to mature and form stabilizing cross-links would be diminished.

The overall picture is of apical tissue (tissues) probably less mature than that found at the mid-root level where collagen bundles are beginning to form. As Zerlotti [61] has indicated such immature tissue is far more susceptible to enzymatic attack. As a consequence the periapical area of young teeth may be particularly responsive to the ravages of tissue break-down products and bacterial toxins carried to it by the lymphatic chan-nels. On the other hand, radicular pulp, having had time to mature, with an increasingly heavy, fibrous collagen component may be more resistant to enzymatic digestion. The final result of these considerations might be what is seen clinically and reported in the literature [25, 33] where radio-graphic evidence of periapical breakdown is manifested in teeth with otherwise reasonably viable pulps.

Pulp Collagen Types

By the late 1970s five distinct collagen molecules had been identified, each with specific α-chain subunits. Type I is almost ubiquitous, but is the main component of bone, dentine, and skin. Type II is typically found in cartilage while type III is present often together with type I in blood vessels, fetal skin, and, of interest here, in distensible tissues such as lung. Base-ment membrane holds most type IV collagen while type V is found in fetal membranes, and as a minor component of bone and cartilage. The reader is referred to other references [6, 12] for further general information.

Perhaps the earliest report of collagen specificity within the pulp was that by Trelstad and Slavkin [55] who found type I but no type IV col-lagen in the primitive dental papilla mesenchyme of the rabbit tooth germ using carboxymethyl cellulose chromatography. In an immunofluorescent study of collagen types in the mouse tooth primordium, Miller and Car-michael [32] located type I in dental papilla and type IV along the entire dentine-enamel junction and in all basement membranes that delineated epithelial-mesenchymal interfaces. Gotoh et al. [15] studied odontogenic cells of the rabbit tooth germ with respect to the synthesis of procollagen

(collagen precursor) types and found that 60% of the secreted precursor was type III procollagen and 40% was type I procollagen.

Using the same animal and technique as Miller and Carmichael [32], Theslaff et al. [53] found only a weak reaction to anticollagen I antibodies in dental mesenchyme during tooth formation; while the reaction to procollagen type III was lost during odontoblastic differentiation, but reappeared with advancing vascularization of the pulp. Takagi [51] utilizing cyanogen bromide digestion of bovine pulp reported that 17% of total collagen was type III. A subsequent investigation [50] found the percentage of type III to increase in bovine pulp from 44% at one year of age to 49% at 4 years of age. Both type I and III were found in bovine dental papilla by Hirschmann and Shuttleworth [23]. In a second paper [47] the amount of type III collagen as a percentage of total collagen increased from 20% in papilla to 31% in pulp (24% papilla, 28% pulp utilizing a different chemical analysis). Leichner and Kalnitsky [29] disputed these results stating that the first study was invalid in so far as human type III collagen was used as a standard. Instead, again using bovine pulp tissue, they [29] found the percentage of type III collagen to remain constant with time at approximately 44%.

Using the ratio of type III to type I as an index Hayakawa et al. [21] found a similar increase in type III in bovine pulp. Whereas the ratio was 0.15 in the partly formed crown stage, by the time of crown attrition from age the ratio had increased to 0.46. In a subsequent article [22] the authors amend these values to 0.13 and 0.32. They also note an increase in the ratio comparing root pulp (0.30) to crown pulp (0.44) for a given tooth.

While most work in this regard has dealt with species other than man, Van Amerongen and Tonino [58], using techniques similar to that of Hayakawa et al. [22], have shown in the human that besides type I collagen a small amount of type III can be found.

In summary it would appear that at least in animal studies (particularly bovine) the two predominent collagen types are I and III and that the percentage of type III may increase with time. The significance of these findings remains speculative, but with the realization that different collagen types exist, an appreciation of changes in tissue distribution and in the quantitative relationships between the two during development became evident. The substitution of one collagen for another and an anatomic redistribution of types may have important consequences for normal function and pathophysiology.

In an effort to correlate the histologic observation of a decrease with age in reticulin (probably type III collagen) to the increasing type III/type I ratio Shuttleworth [47] speculated that perhaps as reticulin decreases, there is a corresponding increase in type III collagen in pulpal blood vessels. Alternatively, type III collagen in the pulp may become associated with type I collagen and consequently lose its argyrophilic nature. The small fibers of 64 nm periodicity noted by Han [17] may represent a combination of type III and type I collagen which together produce a fiber of smaller diameter than type I alone.

Because dentine was believed to contain only type I collagen [11, 23, 44] Leichner and Kalnitsky [29] argued that pulpal collagen fibers containing both type I and type III did not become embedded in dentine as envisaged originally by von Korff [26]. (Other studies report dentine as containing both type I and type III [10, 60]). Part of their argument rested on the fact that collagen content increased in their study from 15 to 24% during development. The authors were in fact measuring collagen concentration (collagen weight/dry weight) rather than collagen content when they state 'total collagen content increases'. As mentioned earlier several studies have shown that pulp collagen content decreases with time [22, 57] while concentration increases.

Theslaff et al. [53] speculated on the significance of type III collagen loss in the mouse tooth germ suggesting that such reduction as has been found in the dental mesenchyme might be one of the features associated with the specificity of the tissue. Furthermore the absence of procollagen type III in the cuspal areas may be associated with cusp formation in tooth morphogenesis.

The increase in type III collagen may be a response of the pulp to an increasingly restrictive environment as a result of root closure and secondary dentine formation [22, 47]. Type III collagen appears in significant amounts in tissues such as skin, aorta, lung, and periodontal ligament where the physiological function of the tissue requires a certain degree of elasticity. It has been suggested that type III collagen presents a compressible cushion allowing for dissipation of intrapulpal pressures arising from inflammation. Van Hassel's [59] finding that an increase in such pressure is a local phenomenon somehow restricted to that area of the pulp adjacent to the toxic stimulus might be interpreted in light of Seltzer et al.'s [46] histologic evidence of coarse collagen fiber bundles walling off the area of inflammation. Perhaps the fibrous wall will be found to contain large amounts of type III collagen and as such represents the pulp's effort to form the cushion necessary to absorb increased inflammatory pressures. Utilizing an immunofluorescent technic it would be interesting to see whether these particular fibers contain higher than usual concentrations of type III collagen.

In conclusion, numerous advances in knowledge regarding pulpal collagen have been made over the past several years. No longer are researchers limited to a more or less descriptive account of the protein's changes with age using the light microscope. Having established a baseline of both quantitative and qualitative changes in the nature of the protein during physiologic aging one can imagine that in the future the more quantifiable techniques seen in this chapter will be applied to st₋ dy the pulp's reaction to the irritants of caries, dental materials, and periodontal disease. The biggest stumbling block may well be the small amount of tissue available in an aged human pulp. It is unfortunate from a research point of view that man does not have bovine teeth with their correspondingly large pulps. Further research may depend on the ability to establish a suitable animal model for testing these parameters.

References

1   Arwill, T.: Studies on the ultrastructure of dental tissues. II. The predentine-pulpal border. Odont. Revy *18:* 191–208 (1967).
2   Avery, J.: Structural elements of the young normal human pulp; in Siskin, The biology of the human dental pulp, pp. 3–15 (Mosby, St. Louis 1973).
3   Avery, J.; Han, S.: Formation of collagen fibrils in the dental pulp. J. dent. Res. *40:* 1248–1261 (1961).
4   Bender, I.; Seltzer, S.; Soltanoff, W.: Endodontic success – a reappraisal of criteria. O.S., O.M., O.P. *22:* 790–802 (1966).
5   Bernick, S.; Nedelman, C.: Effect of aging on the human pulp. J. Endocr. *1:* 88–94 (1975).
6   Bornstein, P.; Sage, H.: Structurally distinct collagen types. A. Rev. Biochem. *49:* 957–1003 (1980).
7   Bhussry, B.: Modification of the dental pulp organ during development and aging; in Finn, Biology of the dental pulp organ, pp. 146–165 (University of Alabama Press, 1968).
8   Breyan, D.; Schilder, H.: An electron microscope study of collagen formation in the dental pulp of the human premolar and rat incisor. Oral Surg. *44:* 437–455 (1977).
9   Childress, R.; Sayegh, F.: Effects of age on pulp ultrastructures (Abstract). J. dent. Res. *58:* 246 (1979).
10 Cournil, I.; Pomponio, J.: Localization of procollagen I and III antigenicity in sections of rat incisor tooth, using the peroxidase-antiperoxidase technique. Anat. Rec. *187:* 557–558 (1977).
11 Dodd, C.; Carmichael, D.: The collagenous matrix of bovine predentin. Biochim. biophys. Acta *577:* 117–182 (1979).
12 Fietzek, P.; Kuhn, K.: The primary structure of collagen. Int. Rev. connect. Tissue Res. *7:* 1–60 (1976).
13 Friend, L.: The treatment of immature teeth with non-vital pulps. J. Br. Endod. Soc. *1:* 28–33 (1967).
14 Gotoh, Y.; Saito, S.; Sato, A.: Synthesis of procollagen by dental pulp cells from incisor in vitro. J. Biochem. *86:* 1037–1040 (1979).
15 Gotoh, Y.; Saito, S.; Sato, A.: Synthesis of procollagen by odontogenic cells of rabbit tooth germ. Biochim. biophys. Acta *587:* 253–262 (1979).
16 Griffin, C.; Harris, R.: Ultrastructure of collagen fibrils and fibroblasts of the developing human dental pulp. Archs oral Biol. *11:* 659–666 (1966).

17 Han, S.: The fine structure of cells and intercellular substances of the dental pulp; in Finn, Biology of the dental pulp organ, pp. 103–144 (University of Alabama Press, 1968).

18 Han, S.; Avery, J.: The fine structure of intercellular substances and rounded cells in the incisor pulp of the guinea pig. Anat. Rec. 151: 41–57 (1965).

19 Han, S.; Avery, J.; Hale, L.: The fine structure of differentiating fibroblasts in the incisor pulp of the guinea pig. Anat. Rec. 153: 187–209 (1965).

20 Harris, R.; Griffin, C.: Histogenesis of fibroblasts in the human dental pulp. Archs oral Biol. 12: 459–468 (1967).

21 Hayakawa, T.; Hashimoto, Y.; Myokei, Y.: Changes in collagen types during the development of bovine dental pulp (Abstract) J. dent. Res. 58: 2279 (1979).

22 Hayakawa, T.; Iijima, K.; Hashimoto, Y.; Myokei, Y.; Takei, T.; Matsui, T.: Developmental changes in the collagens and some collagenolytic activities in bovine dental pulps. Archs oral Biol. 26: 1057–1062 (1981).

23 Hirschmann, P.; Shuttleworth, C.: Collagen heterogeneity in the developing tooth (Abstract). J. dent. Res. 56: D99 (1977).

24 Hubackova, J.; Hornova, J.: The relationship of the dental pulp to age. Oral Res. Abstr. 12: 496 (1977).

25 Jordan, R.; Suzuki, M.; Skinner, D.: Indirect pulp-capping of carious teeth with periapical lesions. J. Am. dent. Ass. 97: 37–43 (1978).

26 Korff, K. von: Die Entwicklung der Zahnbein und Knochengrundsubstanz der Säugetiere. Arch. mikrosk. Anat. Entw Mech. 67: 1–17 (1905).

27 Kuboki, Y.; Takagi, T.; Sasaki, S.; Saito, S.; Mechanic, G.: Comparative collagen biochemistry of bovine periodontium, gingiva, and dental pulp. J. dent. Res. 60: 159–163 (1981).

28 Langeland, K.; Block, R.; Grossman, L.: A histopathologic and histobacteriologic study of 35 periapical endodontic surgical specimens. J. Endocr. 3: 8–12 (1977).

29 Leichner, J.; Kalnitsky, G.: The presence of large amounts of type III collagen in bovine dental pulp and its significance with regard to the mechanism of dentinogenesis. Archs oral Biol. 26: 265–273 (1981).

30 Lin, L. M.; Langeland, K.: Light and electron microscopic study of teeth with carious pulp exposures. Oral Surg. 51: 292–316 (1981).

31 Lin, L.; Shovlin, F.; Skribner, J.; Langeland, K.: Pulp biopsies from the teeth associated with periapical radiolucencies. J. Endocr. 10: 436–448 (1984).

32 Miller, G.; Carmichael, D.: Immunofluorescent localization of collagen types in the mouse primordium (Abstract). J. dent. Res. 58: 382 (1979).

33 Moore, D.: Conservative treatment of teeth with vital pulps and periapical lesions: a preliminary report. J. prosth. Dent. 18: 476–481 (1967).

34 Nielsen, C.; Bentley, J.; Marshall, F.: Age-related changes in reducible crosslinks of human dental pulp collagen. Archs oral Biol. 28: 759–764 (1983).

35 Orlowski, W.: Analysis of collagen, glycoproteins and acid mucopolysaccharides in the bovine and porcine dental pulp. Archs oral Biol. 19: 255–258 (1974).

36 Orlowski, W.: The turnover of collagen in the dental pulp of rat incisors. J. dent. Res. 56: 437–440 (1977).

37 Orlowski, W.: A potential for high collagen turnover in the molar pulp independent of eruption. J. dent. Res. 56: 1488 (1977).

38 Orlowski, W.; Doyle, J.: Collagen metabolism in the pulps of rat teeth. Archs oral Biol. 21: 391–392 (1976).

39 Patten, J.; Jacobs, T.; Hutchins, M.; Turner, S.; Mailman, M.: Collagen synthesis in vitro in developing bovine dental pulp (Abstract). J. dent. Res. 58: 129 (1979).

40 Pearson, C.; Ainsworth, L.: Variations in the hydroxylysyl glycoside contents of collagens in bovine periodontal ligament and dental pulp. J. dent. Res. *57:* 894 (1978).

41 Provenza, D.: The blood vascular supply of the dental pulp with emphasis on capillary circulation. Circulation Res. *6:* 213–218 (1958).

42 Robins, S.; Bailey, A.: The chemistry of the collagen cross-links. The mechanism of stabilization of the reducible intermediate cross-links. Biochem. J. *149:* 381–385 (1975).

43 Robins, S.; Shimokomaki, M.; Bailey, A.: The chemistry of the collagen cross-links. Age-related changes in the reducible components of intact bovine collagen fibers. Biochem. J. *131:* 771–780 (1973).

44 Scott, P.; Veis, A.: The cyanogen bromide peptides of bovine soluble and insoluble collagens. II. Tissue specific crosslinked peptides of insoluble skin and dentin collagen. Connect. Tissue Res. *4:* 117–129 (1976).

45 Seltzer, S.; Bender, I.: The dental pulp, p. 321 (Lippincott, Philadelphia 1975).

46 Seltzer, S.; Bender, I.; Ziontz, M.: The dynamics of pulp inflammation: correlations between diagnostic data and actual histologic findings in the pulp. O.S., O.M., O.P. *16:* 846–871 (1963).

47 Shuttleworth, C.; Ward, J.; Hirschmann, P.: The presence of type III collagen in the developing tooth. Biochim. biophys. Acta *535:* 348–355 (1978).

48 Shuttleworth, C.; Ward, J.; Hirschmann, P.: Extraction of collagen fractions from bovine and rabbit dental follicle, papilla, and pulp. Archs oral Biol. *23:* 235–236 (1978).

49 Stanley, H.; Ranney, R.: Age changes in the human dental pulp. I. The quantity of collagen. O.S., O.M., O.P. *15:* 1396–1404 (1962).

50 Stenstrom, A.; Oreland, L.: Studies of collagen in dental pulps (Abstract). J. dent. Res *58:* 2294 (1979).

51 Takagi, T.: Analysis of collagen cross-links and detection of type III collagen in bovine periodontium, gingiva, and dental pulp. J. Jap. stomatl. Soc. *42:* 42–51 (1975).

52 Takagi, T.; Saito, S.; Kuboki, Y.; Sasaki, S.: Age-related changes of the collagen of periodontium, gingiva, and dental pulp. Jap. J. oral Biol. *17:* 432–441 (1975).

53 Theslaff, I.; Stenman, S.; Vaheri, A.; Timpl. R.: Changes in the matrix proteins, fibronectin and collagen, during differentiation of mouse tooth germ. Dev. Biol. *70:* 116–126 (1979).

54 Toto, P.; Rubinstein, A.; Gargiulo, A.: Labeling index and cell density of aging rat oral tissues. J. dent. Res. *54:* 553–556 (1975).

55 Trelstad, R. L.; Slavkin, H.: Collagen synthesis by the epithelial enamel organ of the embryonic rabbit tooth. Biochem. biophys. Res. Commun. *59:* 443–449 (1974).

56 Uitto, V.; Antila, R.: Characterization of collagen biosynthesis in rabbit dental pulp in vitro. Acta odont. scand. *29:* 609–617 (1971).

57 Uitto, V.; Ranta, R.: Protocollagen proline hydroxylase activity in human dental pulp at various stages of development. Proc. Finn. dent. Soc. *69:* 254–257 (1973).

58 Van Amerongen, J.; Tonino, G.: Collagen in the human pulp (Abstract). J. dent. Res. *58:* 2249 (1979).

59 Van Hassell, H.: Physiology of the human dental pulp. Oral Surg. *32:* 126–134 (1971).

60 Volpin, D.; Veis, A.: Cyanogen bromide peptides from insoluble skin and dentin bovine collagens. Biochemistry, N.Y. *12:* 1452–1464 (1973).

61 Zerlotti, E.: Histochemical study of the connective tissue of the dental pulp. Archs oral Biol. *9:* 149–160 (1964).

Dr. C. J. Nielsen, 5335 Harper Road, Holt, Michigan, Mich. 48842 (USA)

Front. oral Physiol., vol. 6, pp. 126–134 (Karger, Basel 1987)

Saliva Secretion and Composition

Bruce J. Baum

Clinical Investigations and Patient Care Branch, National Institute of Dental Research, National Institutes of Health, Bethesda, Md., USA

Introduction

Any consideration of oral physiology must acknowledge the critical role that saliva plays in oral health. Since the mouth is exposed to the external world, without benefit of many internal defence mechanisms, a unique series of defences are required. Saliva is the principal means by which oral tissues are protected and oral health is maintained. Indeed, the specific functions of saliva in the mouth underlie all normal oral function (table I).

Over the years there has been continuing interest in learning about salivary gland function during aging predominantly due to the anecdotal high prevalence of oral dryness, difficulty in swallowing, diminished taste and tooth loss in elderly persons. Several, but not all, earlier studies supported the notion of decreased (altered) saliva secretion in old age [11, 17, 23, 24, 25] and this conclusion became accepted as an oral physiological fact by many [15, 20, 31]. Relatively recent studies of salivary gland function, however, have suggested that the earlier conclusions were perhaps misleading and that there is no generalized change in salivary gland function during aging [2, 10, 13, 18, 26]. Since previous reports have discussed in detail many reasons for the disparity between earlier and more recent saliva-aging studies [2, 3], it is not necessary to elaborate on these points here. But it is worth noting that these reasons are primarily technical, having to do with less than desirable subject selection and measurement techniques, all of which make data interpretation questionable.

As indicated above, at present we can comfortably conclude that there are no generalized, decremental changes in salivary secretion with increased age in 'healthy' persons. There are certain specific changes which

Table I. Major functions of saliva

Lubrication (mucin, basic proline-rich glycoprotein)
Remineralization (statherin, acidic proline-rich proteins)
Anti-bacterial (sIgA, lysozyme, lactoferrin lactoperoxidase)
Anti-fungal (histidine-rich proteins)
Digestion: food breakdown (amylase, DNase, RNase, proteases)
            food bolus formation (mucin, fluid)
            gustation (fluid, i.e. solvent delivery)
Buffering (bicarbonate, phosphate)

The major functions of saliva are listed and examples of the component(s) which carry out these functions are given in parentheses.

---

have been seen [5]. However, our knowledge of the physiology of salivary glands across the life span is still quite modest. There has been relatively little study of individual gland function, and what exists primarily deals with parotid secretions. Our knowledge of submandibular, sublingual and minor gland saliva secretion and composition is negligible. Accordingly, the present review will, of necessity, emphasize parotid saliva. Although there are many reports utilizing whole saliva, only data related to fluid output will be discussed here. Whole saliva may include, besides saliva constituents, food debris, bacteria and bacterial products, bronchial secretions, desquamated cells and, if there is mucosal compromise, whole blood and serum products [21]. Thus whole saliva constituent data are not necessarily informative about gland function and therefore will not be addressed.

Typically studies on salivary function, as related to a 'clinical situation', often focus on fluid secretion. It should be emphasized that while this facet of gland performance is very important, most of saliva's functions are mediated by specific constituents (usually proteins, see table I). The fluid (water) primarily provides a vehicle delivery and reaction system. We know very little about salivary composition during aging, which by inference means we know little of protein packaging and release by aging human gland cells. Studies with animal models have certainly shown that deficits in protein production can occur with aging [9, 19].

In general, in this chapter, only information obtained with healthy individuals will be discussed. Studies which include clinic/hospital patients, or which are not specific regarding subjects' medical status, are not included because they also present interpretive problems. Similarly studies which have employed inadequate age groupings (e.g. old as 40–99 years vs young as 5–39 years [17]) are not discussed. Finally, it must be

Table II. Parotid saliva flow in different aged healthy males and females*

	Males			Females	
	Y (13)	*M* (14)	*O* (19)	*Y* (17)	*O* (22)
Resting	0.056 ±0.011	0.047 ±0.012	0.044 ±0.009	0.049 ±0.010	0.045 ±0.009
Stimulated	0.80 ±0.10	0.619 ±0.056	0.843 ±0.10	0.62 ±0.08	0.628 ±0.058
Response ratio (log)	1.23	1.3	1.46	1.27	1.25

*These data are from Heft and Baum [18]. For male Y = ≤ 39 years; M = 40–59 years; O = 60 ≥ years. For females Y = premenopausal, and O = postmenopausal, individuals. Numbers in parentheses = number of persons in each group. Data are reported as the mean ± SEM and are expressed as ml/min-gland.

emphasized that all data evaluated are the results of cross-sectional aging studies. There are no reported data from longitudinal studies of salivary gland function and age. Cross-sectional studies, while convenient, are inherently weaker than longitudinal designs.

Parotid Saliva

Several studies have provided data demonstrating that in different aged healthy persons no diminution is found in parotid fluid flow [2, 13, 16, 18]. In table II representative data from a report by Heft and Baum [18] are given. It is clear that both resting and stimulated salivary flow from parotid glands do not change across age groups. Both average values, and the variability in these values, are comparable. Also shown in table II is an index of the degree of responsiveness of glands to stimulation (here 2% citrate swabbed on the tongue dorsum), termed response ratio. This is the log of the value obtained by dividing stimulated flow by unstimulated flow. There is no diminution in the degree of responsiveness to citrate stimulation in parotid glands of older persons.

Gustatory cues, like citrate, are primarily thought to elicit salivation by reflex parasympathetic stimulation of acinar cells [21]. Water transport occurs only through these cells [32] and is now felt to be driven by Cl^- fluxes unidirectionally across basolateral and apical membranes [12,

Table III. General summary of stimulated parotid gland function with increased age

Study	Flow	Na$^+$	K$^+$	Cl$^-$	Protein	Amylase	aPRP	Reference
1	=	↓	=	↓	↓	=	n.d.	13
2	=	↓	=	n.d.	=	n.d.	=	7, 8

In both studies healthy, community dwelling persons were examined (study 1, males; study 2, males + females). aPRP refers to the anionic proline-rich proteins, a known constituent of serous acinar cell secretory granules. n.d. = Not done.

14, 22]. The flow rate data available with the aging parotid gland imply that this fluid driving mechanism (which includes muscarinic receptor coupling, a basolateral Na$^+$/K$^+$/Cl$^-$ cotransporter, and an apical Ca^{2-} dependent Cl$^-$ channel) 'normally' remains intact throughout the human life span.

At present there are no data available on the composition of unstimulated parotid saliva. Two laboratories have, however, reported compositional information on stimulated parotid secretions [7, 8, 13]. A summary of their findings is given in table III, while actual values for certain important constituents are given in table IV. In general, the findings between the two laboratories are in reasonable agreement. The central observations include a diminution in Na$^+$ content, no change in K$^+$ output and no change in acinar secretory protein release (amylase and anionic proline-rich proteins, a PRP) of saliva obtained from older persons.

What do such compositional data infer about gland function? First, the Na$^+$ data probably indicate increased Na$^+$ reabsorption by duct cells in glands from older persons. This is particularly obvious when Na$^+$ data are viewed in conjunction with salivary flow rates [7]. Saliva originates as an isotonic primary secretion and Na$^+$ is reabsorbed to a considerable extent in the striated duct section in a flow rate-related manner [32]. For some reason, as yet unclear, older persons conserve more Na$^+$ by this process [7]. K$^+$, originally at low levels in primary saliva ($\sim$5 mM), is secreted by ductal cells resulting in final gland saliva [K$^+$] of typically $\sim$15–20 mM. It is not known by what transport mechanism K$^+$ is secreted (or for that matter, exactly how Na$^+$ is reabsorbed). But the data clearly show there is no impairment in K$^+$ release by duct cells in parotid glands of older persons. Finally, the observations on amylase and aPRP release suggest that there is no general impairment in exocrine protein production, packaging into secretory granules, or exocytotic release by parotid acinar cells with age. In aggregate, such findings and conclusions support

Table IV. Representative constituent levels in stimulated parotid saliva of different aged healthy males and females

	Y	M	O
Males			
[Na+]1, mEq/l	30.3 ± 3.1	21.7 ± 2.8	20.3 ± 2.4
[K+]1, mEq/l	16.4 ± 1.4	17.8 ± 0.5	18.2 ± 0.6
Protein2, mg/ml	3.22 ± 0.34	2.74 ± 0.21	2.67 ± 0.18
aPRP output2, mg/min	0.43 ± 0.06	0.42 ± 0.11	0.41 ± 0.05
Females			
[Na+]1, mEq/l	34.3 ± 4.1	26.0 ± 4.1	30.1 ± 3.6
[K+]1, mEq/l	18.2 ± 0.5	17.3 ± 0.7	19.1 ± 0.7
Protein2, mg/ml	3.03 ± 0.25	3.24 ± 0.30	3.07 ± 0.36
aPRP output2, mg/min	0.49 ± 0.12	0.49 ± 0.11	0.50 ± 0.08

[1] These date were previously reported [7] and represent of mean ± SEM of measurements from 38–44 males of 24–28 females per age group. Y = ≤ 39 years; M = 40–59 years; O = ≥ 60 years.
[2] These data were previously reported [8] and represent in mean ± SEM of measurement from 29–37 males or 14–18 females per age group (same as above).

the contention that there is no overall decrement in parotid gland function during aging. This stands in contrast to earlier findings of descriptive morphological changes occurring with age in the human parotid gland [1]. Apparently the morphological changes must be either functionally insignificant or influencing only a proportionally minimal amount of gland parenchyma. Although many of the components of parotid saliva which play important roles in oral health (table I) have not been studied with respect to aging, the spectrum of performance characteristics examined thus far are consistent with a concept that the human parotid gland is an example of an exocrine tissue which remains functionally intact across the human life span.

Submandibular and Minor Gland Saliva

As stated earlier, there exists very little information on the performance of other human salivary glands with aging. To date, there is only one reported study each on submandibular (accurately submandibular/sublingual) and minor gland (labial) salivas. These studies, both from the same laboratory, examined only fluid secretion by these glands [16, 27].

Table V. Submandibular and labial minor gland flow rates in different aged persons

	Resting		Stimulated	
	Y	O	Y	O
Submandibular	0.058 ± 0.009	0.013 ± 0.004	0.264 ± 0.25	0.103 ± 0.017
	(28)	(26)	(30)	(28)
Labial minor	n.d.	n.d.	2.85 ± 0.23	1.34 ± 0.26
			(12)	(13)

Data for submandibular flow is from Pedersen et al. [27] and are the mean ± SEM, expressed as ml/min/gland. For this study Y = 18–35 years while 0 = ≥ 66 years. Data for labial minor flow are from Gandara et al. [16] and are the mean ± SEM, expressed as μl/min. For this study Y = < 59 years while O = ≥ 59 years. Numbers in parentheses = number of persons in each group. n.d. = Not determined.

A summary of these data is shown in table V. For each secretion tested, older individuals showed a significantly lower flow rate than was obtained with younger persons.

It is of particular interest to note that despite the lower resting flow rate seen from submandibular glands of older persons, the glands respond well to stimulation (the percent increase is greater in the older individuals than the younger ones). Previously Waterhouse et al. [33] and Scott [28, 29] have reported morphometric data showing that there is a significant reduction in acinar parenchymal tissue (~40–50%) with increased age in human submandibular glands. One can speculate that since the fluid driving force originates in acinar cells [32], the reduction in flow rates observed by Pedersen et al. [27] is coupled to this morphologic change. The situation occurring with the aging submandibular gland thus raises interesting questions regarding the relationship between gland mass, fluid flow and functional reserve capacity. A good deal more study is required however before any firm conclusions can be drawn.

There is a similar need to obtain information on the composition of submandibular and minor gland salivas from different aged persons. This is particularly acute with respect to the unique protein products of mucous acinar cells, the mucins. Mucins are apparently the key lubricatory molecules in the oral cavity (table I), playing an important role in maintaining the mucosal barrier function and facilitating food bolus formation and swallowing. They may contribute as well to the sensation of oral wetness. There is evidence in the rat submandibular gland for a relatively specific perturbation in mucin production and processing with increased age [9].

Table VI. Summary of whole saliva fluid output with increased age

	Resting	Stimulated
Males	↓	=
Females	↓	=

These conclusions are based on reports by Bertram [11] Parvinen and Larmas [26] and Ben-Aryeh et al. [10] and represent populations in Denmark, Finland and Israel, respectively. Gandara et al. [16], studying a population in the USA, found no changes in different aged persons in both resting and simulated whole saliva fluid output.

Whole Saliva

There are very few conclusions concerning aging glandular function which can be made from studying whole saliva. Yet it is clear that the vast majority of fluid detected in the mouth (except perhaps in the case of persons with severe gland damage and marked oral mucositis) is in large part a result of gland parenchymal water transport. Several investigators have examined whole saliva fluid output in different aged healthy persons. A summary of findings is presented in table VI. Two separate studies have shown decreased resting whole saliva flow in older persons [10, 11] and one study has shown no change [16]. Three studies have all shown no change in stimulated fluid output [10, 16, 26].

The notion of a decreased amount of whole saliva present basally is consistent with findings noted above for submandibular gland secretions. Given that glands of older persons respond well to secretory stimuli, it is not surprising that age differences in fluid output may disappear after stimulation. The inconsistencies observed between studies may reflect the techniques used to collect 'resting' whole saliva (certainly true basal levels of whole saliva would be difficult to measure), as well as different characteristics in the study populations. In general though, older persons who are healthy have readily measurable levels of fluid in their mouths. If, as in the case of resting whole saliva, statistically significant differences exist between young and old persons, we must not rush to conclude that such differences are also biologically significant.

Concluding Remarks

At the onset of this chapter, many boundaries were stated which in effect served to limit the amount of material presented. These limitations are realistic considerations for any critical discussion of the normal physiology of salivary secretion across the life span. The inevitable conclusion is that there simply are not sufficiently abundant data available on saliva secretion and composition to generate an extensive discussion of the subject. There is considerable need to collect more data, especially with submandibular/sublingual and minor gland secretions. Despite the given limitations, this chapter has clearly shown that diminished salivary gland performance, once considered a fact of geriatric oral health, is better viewed as a myth. Changes in oral health, which may accompany aging and which are suggestive of altered salivary secretion, are more likely due to disease and its pharmacologic treatment [4, 6, 30].

References

1   Andrew, W. A.: A comparison of age changes in salivary glands of man and of the rat. J. Gerontol. 7: 178–190 (1952).
2   Baum, B. J.: Evaluation of stimulated parotid saliva flow rate in different age groups. J. dent. Res. 60: 1292–1296 (1981).
3   Baum, B. J.: Research on aging and oral health: an assessment of current status and future needs. Spec. Care Dent. 1: 156–165 (1981).
4   Baum, B. J.: Normal and abnormal oral status in aging. A. Rev. Gerontol. Geriat. 4: 87–105 (1984).
5   Baum, B. J.: Salivary gland function during aging. Gerodontics 2: 61–64 (1986).
6   Baum, B. J.; Bodner, L.; Fox, P. C.; Izutsu, K. T.; Pizzo, P.; Wright, W. E.: Therapy-induced dysfunctions of salivary glands. Spec. Care Dent. 5: 274–277 (1985).
7   Baum, B. J.; Costa, P. T., Jr.; Izutsu, K. T.: Sodium handling by aging human parotid glands is inconsistent with two-stage secretion model. Am. J. Physiol. 246: R35–R39 (1984).
8   Baum, B. J.; Kousvelari, E. E.; Oppenheim, F. G.: Exocrine protein secretion from human parotid glands during aging: stable release of the acidic proline-rich proteins. J. Geront. 37: 392–395 (1982).
9   Baum, B. J.; Kuyatt, B. L.; Humphreys, S.: Protein production and processing in young adult and aged rat submandibular gland cells in vitro. Mech. Age. Dev. 23: 123–136 (1983).
10 Ben-Aryeh, H.; Miron, D.; Szargel, R.; Gutman, D.: Whole saliva secretion rates in old and young healthy subjects. J. dent. Res. 63: 1147–1148 (1984).
11 Bertram, U.: Xerostomia. Acta odont. scand. 25: suppl. 49 (1967).
12 Case, R. M.; Hunter, M.; Novak, I.; Young, J. A.: The anionic basis of fluid secretion by the rabbit mandibular salivary gland. J. Physiol., Lond. 349: 619–630 (1984).
13 Chauncey, H. H.; Borkan, G.; Wayler, A.; Feller, R. P.; Kapur, K. K.: Parotid fluid composition in healthy aging males. Adv. Physiol. Sci. 28: 323–328 (1981).
14 Findlay, I.; Peterson, O. H.: Acetylcholine stimulates a Ca^{2+}-dependent Cl^- conductance in mouse lacrimal acinar cells. Pflugers Arch. 403: 328–330 (1985).
15 Franks, A. S. T.; Hedegaard, B.: Geriatric dentistry (Blackwell, Oxford 1973).
16 Gandara, B. K.; Izutsu, K. T.; Truelove, E. L.; Ensign, W. Y.; Sommers, E. E.: Age-related salivary flow rate changes in controls and patients with oral lichen planus. J.

dent. Res. *64:* 1149–1151 (1985).

17   Grad, B.: Diurnal, age and sex changes in sodium and potassium concentration of whole saliva. J. Geront. *9:* 276–280 (1954).

18   Heft, M. W.; Baum, B. J.: Unstimulated and stimulated parotid salivary flow rate in individuals of different ages. J. dent. Res. *63:* 1182–1185 (1984).

19   Kim, S. K.; Calkins, D. W.: Secretory protein synthesis in parotid glands of young and old rats. Archs oral Biol. *28:* 1–4 (1983).

20   Langer, A.: Oral signs of aging and their clinical significance. Geriatrics *31:* 63–69 (1976).

21   Mandel, I. D.: Sialochemistry in disease and clinical situations affecting salivary glands. CRC crit. Rev. clin. Lab. Sci. *12:* 321–366 (1980).

22   Martinez, J. R.; Cassity, N.: Effect of transport inhibitors on secretion by perfused rat submandibular gland. Am. J. Physiol. *245:* G711–G716 (1983).

23   Mason, D. K.; Chisholm, D. M.: Salivary glands in health and disease (Saunders, London 1975).

24   Meyer, J.; Necheles, H.: Studies in old age. IV. The clinical significance of salivary, gastric and pancreatic secretion in the aged. J. Am. med. Ass. *115:* 2050–2055 (1940).

25   Meyer, J.; Spier, E.; Neuwalt, F.: Basal secretion of digestive enzymes in old age. Archs intern. Med. *65:* 171–177 (1940).

26   Parivinen, T.; Larmas, M.: Age dependency of stimulated salivary flow rate, pH and lactobacillus and yeast concentrations. J. dent. Res. *61:* 1052–1055 (1982).

27   Pedersen, W.; Schubert, M.; Izutsu, K.; Mersai, T.; Truelove, E.: Age-dependent decreases in human submandibular gland flow rates as measured under resting and post-stimulation conditions. J. dent. Res. *64:* 822–825 (1985).

28   Scott, J.: Quantitative age changes in the histological structure of human submandibular salivary glands. Archs oral Biol. *22:* 221–227 (1977).

29   Scott, J.: A morphometric study of age changes in the histology of the ducts of human submandibular glands. Archs oral Biol. *22:* 243–249 (1977).

30   Sreebny, L. M.; Schwartz, S. S.: A reference guide to drugs and dry mouth. Gerodontology *5:* 75–99 (1986).

31   Storer, R.: The oral tissues; in Brocklehurst, Textbook of geriatric medicine and gerontology, pp. 330–340 (Churchill-Livingstone, London 1978).

32   Young, J. A.; Lennep, E. W. van: Transport in salivary and salt glands; in Giebisch, Tosteson, Ussing, Membrane transport in biology, pp. 563–674 (Springer, Berlin 1979).

33   Waterhouse, J. P.; Chisholm, D. M.; Winter, R. B.; Patel, M.; Yale, R. S.: Replacement of functional parenchymal cells by fat and connective tissue in human salivary glands: an age-related change. J. oral Pathol. *2:* 16–27 (1973).

Dr. B. J. Baum, Clinical Investigations and Patient Care Branch, National Institute of Dental Research, Building 10, Room 1A–06, Bethesda, MD 20892 (USA)

Front. oral Physiol., vol. 6, pp. 135–150 (Karger, Basel 1987)

Aging and Chemosensory Perception

Claire Murphy[1]

San Diego State University, Department of Psychology, San Diego, Calif., USA

Introduction

An implicit or explicit interest in nutrition in the elderly has recently generated an increased interest in studies of chemosensory function in the elderly. Although evidence is mounting to support the existence of decline in function with age, research has focused primarily on threshold measurement and, more recently, on suprathreshold intensity function. The question of altered chemosensory preference has largely escaped direct address.

Threshold studies of the gustatory system have demonstrated modest increases in threshold with age [1, 4, 9, 12, 17, 18, 19, 20, 21, 22, 23, 26, 27, 30, 35, 37, 42, 46, 47, 49, 51, 52, 58]. Although some authors have reported quality-specific changes with aging [59] none of the four basic tastes (sweet, sour, salty, or bitter) has escaped report of age-related decline by at least one investigator. There is currently some debate regarding both the magnitude of the decline and its role in perception of real-world stimuli.

Recent studies have investigated age-related changes in suprathreshold taste intensity perception [see ref. 42 for a review]. Enns et al. [15] found no alteration in the slope of the psychophysical function for taste from young adulthood to old age, although slopes for two adult groups (both 1.12) were flatter than the slope for fifth graders (1.72). Bartoshuk [2] has reported stability of slopes in the elderly, but sees some flattening near threshold which she attributes to lack of dental hygiene. Schiffman and Clark [48], Schiffman et al. [51], and Cowart [10] all re-

[1] The author's research and the preparation of this article was supported by NIH Grant No. AG04085 from the National Institute on Aging. I am grateful to Maggie Jensen, Elizabeth Konowal, Carol Randall, Michele J. Reed and Jeanne Withee for excellent technical assistance.

ported some flattening of the slopes of taste functions in elderly subjects, suggesting some decline in the ability of the elderly to track increases in a stimulus concentration.

In the real world, perception of stimuli in the oral cavity most often involves not only taste information (i.e. information about sweet, sour, bitter and salty), but also olfactory and trigeminal information from the myriad of volatiles in foods and beverages. Independent of age-associated taste differences, age-related differences in the backdrop of volatiles accompanying a taste may influence its perception, particularly its pleasantness. Olfactory threshold studies have yielded almost unanimous agreement that there is age-related decline, both for stimuli which are largely olfactory, and for stimuli which are largely trigeminal [8, 16, 25, 28, 33, 40, 45, 50, 56, 57; see ref. 42 for a review]. Age-related deficits in intensity perception of suprathreshold olfactory and trigeminal stimuli have now also been demonstrated [38, 40, 41, 54, 55]. In most cases the up-down position of the psychophysical function was affected, in others the slope of the function.

Given substantial evidence suggesting both threshold and supra-threshold age-related differences in sensitivity of the chemical senses, the question arises: How is preference for chemosensory stimuli affected by age? What scant literature addresses this question does not completely answer it.

Taste Preferences in Subjects of Different Ages

Laird and Breen [29] reported an increased preference for tart taste over sweet taste in older subjects and to a lesser degree in females of all ages.

Although Desor et al. [11] demonstrated that, in a sample of 618 children and 140 adults, 9- to 15-year-olds preferred greater sweetness and saltiness than did adults 18–64 years old; no additional age effects emerged when preferences of adults 18–29 years and 45–64 years were compared. The proportions of the adult group falling into these age ranges were not reported.

Enns et al. [15] measured preferences for sucrose in 21 fifth graders, 27 college students, and 12 elderly subjects, and found that fifth graders and the elderly females showed a lesser preference for sweeter sucrose solutions than did the college age participants and males of all ages. Dye and Koziatek [12] measured pleasantness of suprathreshold aqueous solutions of sucrose for 79 diabetic and non-diabetic veterans. When pleasantness judgments of men 41–65 years were compared with those of men

65–88 years, the three-way interaction of age, patient group, and sucrose level was significant at the 0.0001 level. Older non-diabetic subjects increased pleasantness ratings over the range 0.125–1 M. Younger non-diabetic subjects rated 0.25 M as the pleasantest and decreased their pleasantness ratings with each subsequent concentration.

Age-related preference differences in the amount of salt added to chicken broth were found by Braddock and Pangborn [unpublished data]. Older (36- to 66-year-old) subjects added more salt than younger (17- to 32-year-old) subjects when allowed to salt to preference.

Age-related odor preference shifts were shown by Engen [13, 14] and Moncrieff [34]. Mere exposure to odors [7] or to olfactory-taste mixtures, presented orally, can produce shifts in pleasantness [39]. Murphy [39] also demonstrated effects of context on the pleasantness of chemosensory stimuli. Exposure-related pleasantness shifts occurring over a lifetime could result in altered food and odor preferences in the elderly.

Preference shifts need not necessarily be correlated with an underlying alteration in the sensory system. However, a change in the ability of a chemosensory system to process intensity information, reflected in a change in slope or up-down position of the psychophysical functions, would predict a change in preferred concentration and hedonic judgments, since intensity has been shown to be a powerful predictor of hedonic tone [36]. If, for example, the salty function flattened with age, then a stimulus which is too salty for a young person will be less salty for an elderly person and may move from negative to positive in hedonic tone.

When considering the question of chemosensory hedonics, it is useful to make a distinction between preference and pleasantness. Two useful measures of hedonics are the peak preferred concentration (i.e. that one concentration in a series which is chosen as the most preferred) and the pleasantness judgment (i.e. a kind of magnitude estimate of the pleasantness or unpleasantness of a given stimulus). These two measures provide different types of information concerning the hedonic quality of a stimulus. The former identifies the most preferred stimulus concentration in a series and the latter provides information about the pleasantness of each stimulus in the series. Both measures may be important in assessing age-associated changes in chemosensory hedonics. For example, in a series of four concentrations of sucrose, young and elderly subjects might both choose the third concentration as the most preferred. However, the elderly might rate the fourth and highest concentration as pleasant while the young subjects might rate the sweetest stimulus as unpleasant. For this reason the study described below was designed to yield information regarding the existence of age-associated differences in both of these measures.

Age-Related Changes in Preferences as Affected by
Concentration and Presentation of Stimuli

After reviewing the literature investigating the relationship of age
and chemosensory preference, it was obvious that a large-scale study of
taste preference across the adult life span was lacking. Therefore, the
author designed a large cross-sectional study to investigate the existence
of age-related changes in preference for various concentrations of single
tastants and of the same tastants in more complex chemosensory mixtures. Complete details regarding this study will be found in Murphy and
Withee [43]. Several questions were addressed. First, does the concentration most preferred in a series differ over the life span for the stimuli salt,
sugar or citric acid? Second, are there age-associated changes in pleasantness judgments for various concentrations of salt, sugar or citric acid?
Third, does the background in which a stimulus is presented significantly
affect the hedonic tone of that stimulus?

Of the 300 persons tested, 100 were young adults with a mean age of
21 years, 100 were middle-aged adults with a mean age of 37 years and
100 were older adults with a mean age of 73 years.

The stimuli were sucrose, citric acid and NaCl, each presented in four
concentrations in deionized water and the same four concentrations in
appropriate beverage bases. Preference was measured on a bipolar line
scale where marks to the left of zero indicated unpleasantness, marks to
the right of zero indicated pleasantness and marks through zero indicated
hedonic neutrality. Distance from zero reflected the magnitude of
pleasantness or unpleasantness. Pleasantness judgments were normalized
according to Murphy [39].

A four-way (age, stimulus, background, concentration) analysis of
variance (ANOVA) on the pleasantness ratings showed significant effects
of age, background, stimulus and concentration. Mean pleasantness ratings were less negative for elderly participants than for either young
or middle-aged participants. Stimuli were judged less pleasant overall
in an aqueous base than in a beverage base and concentration significantly affected ratings. The significant interactions of age with stimulus,
background with stimulus and of age, stimulus and concentration
provide interesting insights into age-associated differences in pleasantness. Young and middle-aged participants found salt significantly less
pleasant than did elderly subjects. Similarly, the mean pleasantness
ratings for sucrose were significantly higher for older subjects than for
middle-aged, but not for young subjects. The two highest concentrations of sucrose were also rated as pleasanter by the elderly participants
than by the younger participants. Citric was less pleasant than NaCl

for elderly subjects, but the reverse was true for young and middle-aged subjects.

Pleasantness judgments of all three stimuli were significantly affected by the background base in which they were presented. Sucrose and NaCl were both rated more pleasant in the beverage base, but the background produced greater differences in the pleasantness of NaCl than in the pleasantness of sucrose. Salt was rated as pleasanter by the elderly than by other participants regardless of its background. When presented in deionized water, increasing NaCl concentration drove pleasantness down for all age groups. However, when presented in beverage base, the two middle salt concentrations were preferred to the lowest by both middle-aged and elderly raters. Citric acid was perceived as less pleasant in the beverage base than in the aqueous base.

Figure 1 shows the differential responses of the three age groups to the three stimuli.

As figure 2 illustrates, the background base in which they were presented significantly affected the pleasantness judgments of all three stimuli, for sucrose (all means differ with $p < 0.01$).

The interaction of age with stimulus and concentration is shown in figure 3. Figure 3 also shows, across the three age groups, that while pleasantness ratings generally decrease for both NaCl and citric acid, the ratings for sucrose increase for the first three concentrations, dropping at the fourth to produce inverted U-shaped functions.

Similarly, elderly subjects rated the two highest concentrations of sucrose as pleasanter than the lowest concentration, and they rated them more pleasant than the younger subjects did.

The data were analyzed for peak preferred concentration by a three-factor (age, background, stimulus) ANOVA with repeated measures. Results showed that the peak preferred concentration differed as a function of background and of stimulus. The mean preferred concentration was higher in beverage base than in aqueous solution. Regardless of background, participants preferred higher concentrations of sucrose than of NaCl or citric acid. This relatively gross measure did not capture the age effect seen in the analysis of the individual pleasantness ratings.

The findings of this study have implications for dietary intake in elderly people, particularly those who must restrict their intake of salt and sugar. Elderly people as a group have increased incidence of hypertension and diabetes. There is also a gradual rise in systolic blood pressure with age which may have clinical sequelae which are as yet not known or understood. Similarly, there is a general tendency for blood sugar to rise with age and the clinical implications of this are not entirely clear.

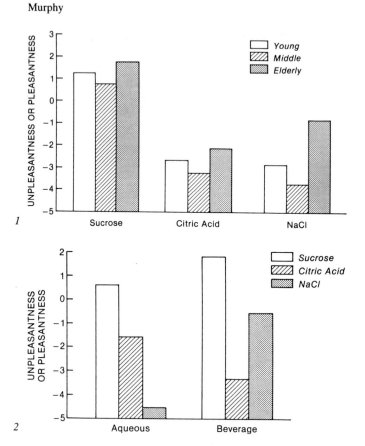

Fig. 1. Mean pleasantness or unpleasantness ratings of sucrose, citric acid, and NaCl by young, middle-aged, and elderly subjects. From Murphy and Withee [43].

Fig. 2. Mean pleasantness or unpleasantness ratings of sucrose, citric acid, and NaCl shown as rated in aqueous solution and in the beverage bases. From Murphy and Withee [43].

Both diet and exercise have been shown to be beneficial in controlling blood pressure and blood glucose levels [6, 31, 32]. Compliance to diet regimes is difficult at any age, but can be particularly difficult for elderly persons. Decreased energy expenditure results in decreased caloric needs and therefore reduced intake is necessary to maintain energy balance. Since many elderly persons must restrict intake of salt and sugar for medical reasons, taste preference for these stimuli can be important for the health of the elderly population.

High concentrations of sucrose and NaCl were rated as pleasanter by elderly than by younger participants. The most obvious possible explana-

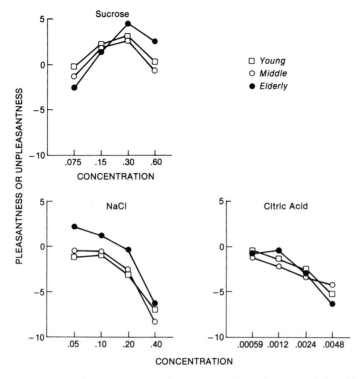

Fig. 3. Mean pleasantness or unpleasantness ratings of sucrose, citric acid and NaCl shown as a function of age and of concentration. From Murphy and Withee [43]. Copyright by the American Psychological Association.

tion for this effect appears to be sensory. Older people may, for example, rate higher concentrations of salt as pleasanter simply because these concentrations are less salty to them than to younger subjects who generally rate very high concentrations of salt as unpleasant. The fact that some investigators have reported a flattening of the slopes for psychophysical functions for some of the simple tastants [10] and for amino acids [48] in the elderly lends some support to this sensory hypothesis. However, since the above-mentioned studies used the magnitude estimation technique, no information regarding absolute differences in intensity was obtained. The results of the present study do suggest that an experiment designed to directly test the ability of intensity to predict chemosensory hedonics across the life-span would be worthwhile.

As with any cross-sectional aging study the question of cohort differences in the present study arises. Environmental influences may have interacted with sensory influences on perception of flavor. The significant age effects on pleasantness ratings in the present study suggest the importance of future longitudinal studies.

The fact that pleasantness judgments shift when when the taste stimuli are in beverage base versus aqueous base underscores the importance of other chemosensory elements in determining pleasantness. Age-associated changes in olfactory perception may be partially responsible for the differences in pleasantness judgments made by the young, middle-aged and elderly subjects in these experiments. An older person might, for instance, rate a stronger concentration of salt in the beverage base as more pleasant, not necessarily because he desired more intense taste per se, but because he desired an overall stronger flavor. He or she could compensate for reduced sensory input from volatiles by increasing sensory input to the taste system. Experiments considering the ability of elderly and young subjects to identify blended food, with and without the sense of smell, clearly demonstrated that the olfactory system was more affected by the aging process than the taste system [38, 41]. Others have since come to the same conclusion [54].

The importance of the diluent in chemosensory preference research was clear from this study. Research investigating pleasantness of stimuli in aqueous solution may not present a clear picture of real-world preferences of humans. Sodium chloride in water and sucrose in water are not generally consumed in the USA. On the average, subjects in the present study chose as their most preferred a concentration of NaCl in vegetable juice which exceeded their preferred concentration in deionized water. This result seems to be related to subjects' clear preference for salt in foods and beverages naturally consumed, in spite of their distaste for concentrated solutions of salt in water. In the past, many studies of taste preference have been conducted with deionized water or distilled water as the diluent. The generalizability of results with pure tastants such as NaCl and sucrose in water to real world preference for salt and sugar needs to be reassessed.

Elderly people find salt and sugar pleasanter at higher concentrations than younger subjects do. The reasons for this may be cultural, contextural or sensory. An investigation of chemosensory preference and chemosensory intensity simultaneously in a single group of elderly and young persons will be an important next step in the process of understanding the effects of the aging process on chemosensory perception and pleasantness.

Nutritional Status and Taste Sensation

Recent biochemical studies have reported significant nutritional deficits in samples of elderly people. Though it remains unclear whether these nutritional deficiencies result from decreased nutrient intake [5 for a review, see ref. 3], or from lowered rates of absorption and utilization in the elderly [60], or from a combination of factors, the problem appears to be widespread. Studies by Yearick et al. [60] and Jansen and Harrill [24] report that up to 41% of elderly participants show deficient levels of serum protein, and 20% show deficiency in serum albumin.

Although many of the recent studies of the chemical senses in aged people have been conducted with the implicit or explicit assumption that age-associated changes in chemosensory perception are related to health and nutritional status in elderly persons, experimental evidence to back this assumption is lacking.

Investigation of Effects of Nutritional Status: Experiment 1

The research described below was designed to investigate a clear-cut link between nutritional status and chemosensory preference in elderly persons. A complete description of these experiments may be found in Murphy and Withee [44]. Nutritional status was operationally defined as the biochemical indices of total protein, albumin, and blood urea nitrogen (BUN).

We first investigated the effects of aging and biochemical status on preference for casein hydrolysate, an amino acid mixture. The hypotheses were that (a) older participants would rate high concentrations of the amino acid mixture as more pleasant than young participants would, and (b) that participants with lower biochemical status would prefer higher concentrations of casein hydrolysate than would those with better biochemical status.

Method

The participants were 10 persons 18–26 years old ($M = 22.8$) and 16 persons 70–92 years of age ($M = 84.0$). The young participants were students and technicians, and the elderly participants were recruited from senior centers and senior citizen's apartment complexes in an urban area.

The chemosensory stimuli consisted of an amino acid-deficient soup base to which were added the following concentrations of casein hydrolysate: 0, 1, 2, 3, 4, and 5% weight per volume. Stimuli were prepared in deionized water, refrigerated, and then heated before presentation.

The participants rated pleasantness of the chemosensory stimuli using a bipolar line scale described above for the previous study. Blood was drawn from each person, usually on the same day, and an independent laboratory provided an assay of serum total protein, albumin, and BUN.

Results

Elderly participants had, on the average, higher BUN and lower albumin and protein values. Of the 16 elderly participants, 7 had low serum protein levels, defined as less than 6.5 g/dl. One young participant had a protein level less than 6.5 g/dl.

An analysis of variance was performed to examine the effect of age on peak preferred concentration (PPC), which was defined as the concentration (0, 1, 2, 3, 4, or 5% casein hydrolysate) most preferred by each participant. Results, presented in figure 4, showed that older participants preferred higher concentrations of casein hydrolysate ($M = 3.0\%$) than did young participants ($M = 0.5\%$).

Similar analyses examining the effect of the three blood measures (grouped above and below the median) on PPC showed higher concentrations of casein hydrolysate were preferred by those with higher values of BUN, and those with lower serum albumin (fig. 5). There was no difference in preferred concentration associated with serum protein level.

Investigation of Effects of Nutritional Status: Experiment 2

These results suggested, in a small sample, the influence of age and biochemical status on the perceived plesantness of casein hydrolysate. A second experiment was designed to further investigate these variables as well as to determine the effect of perceived intensity on preference for casein hydrolysate. There were three hypotheses (1) that older participants would prefer higher concentrations of the amino acid mixture, (2) that participants of lower biochemical status would prefer higher concentrations of casein hydrolysate, and (3) that perceived intensity would be predictive of preference.

Method

Of the 40 participants in this study, 20 were 18–26 years of age ($M = 20.15$) and the remaining 20 were 65–83 years of age ($M = 70.75$). Each age group contained 7 men and 13 women who were active, community-dwelling persons with no hospitalizations in the preceding 12 months.

The method of magnitude matching, modulus-free developed by Stevens and Marks [53], which embodies elements of both magnitude estimation and cross-modality matching,

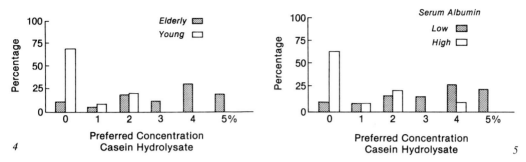

Fig. 4. Peak preferred concentration of the amino acid mixture as a function of age (first experiment). From Murphy and Withee [44].

Fig. 5. Peak preferred concentration of the amino acid mixture as a function of albumin status. From Murphy and Withee [44].

was used to determine intensity of the same six chemosensory stimuli used in the first experiment as well as of six auditory stimuli which were included only for the purposes of matching. Participants assigned numbers on the same scale of magnitude to reflect perceived intensity of both the auditory stimuli and the chemosensory stimuli.

Participants also rated pleasantness of both auditory and chemosensory stimuli using the bipolar line scale described above. Marks to the left of the zero midpoint indicated unpleasantness and marks to the right of zero indicated pleasantness. The distance from the zero midpoint represented the degree of unpleasantness or pleasantness.

Results

Biochemical Indices. Comparison of the mean values for the three biochemical indices for young and elderly participants showed that there were significant age group differences in biochemical status for all three measures. Elderly participants showed lower levels of serum protein and albumin, and elevated levels of BUN compared to young participants. 20% of the elderly had low serum protein levels (below 6.5 g/dl). None of the young participants had low or deficient levels of protein. For the remaining analyses a composite of the three blood measures was created by combining each subject's standard (z) scores (protein + albumin – BUN). The resulting index represented a subject's biochemical status.

Intensity. Chemosensory intensity judgments were normalized by auditory intensity judgments, using a procedure described by Stevens et al. [55] before being subjected to ANOVA. Age group and concentration significantly affected intensity estimates. Older participants made lower-intensity estimates for amino acids (geometric mean = 3.3) than did young participants (geometric mean = 5.4), all participants successfully tracked increases in concentration. Age group differences in intensity were similar at all concentrations of casein hydrolysate.

The lack of a significant interaction in the ANOVA implied that there was no age effect on the slopes of the psychophysical functions produced by the two age groups. Biochemical status showed no significant relationship to perceived intensity.

Peak Preferred Concentration. Experiment 1 indicated that age and the biochemical measures affected participants' PPC of casein hydrolysate. In order to test in an ANOVA these effects and the effect of perceived intensity on the PPC of casein hydrolysate, a geometric mean intensity rating was computed for each participant across the six concentrations. Since, as previously reported, biochemical measures and intensity estimates were different for young and elderly, for this analysis both the geometric mean intensity rating and the previously described composite biochemical index were grouped above and below appropriate age group medians.

A three-way ANOVA showed that age and blood status (as measured by the biochemical index described above) were significantly related to PPC, but perceived intensity was not. Elderly participants preferred higher concentrations of casein hydrolysate ($M = 1.4\%$) than did young participants ($M = 0.4\%$). Across age, participants with lower composite biochemical indices also preferred higher concentrations of amino acids ($M = 1.5\%$) than participants with higher biochemical status ($M = 0.4\%$).

The percentages of each age group who preferred each of the concentrations of casein hydrolysate showed essentially the same pattern as was found in the first experiment and plotted in figure 4.

Discussion of Experimental Data

Two of the initial hypotheses in experiment 2 were confirmed: (a) older participants preferred higher concentrations of the amino acid mixture, and (b) participants with lower values for the combined biochemical index preferred higher concentrations of the amino acid mixture. Although the elderly participants had lower geometric mean intensity estimates, a participant's overall mean perceived intensity did not predict his preference. Thus, these present studies revealed individual differences in preference for a nutritionally significant chemosensory stimulus, which varied independently with both biochemical status and age.

It is, of course, interesting to speculate upon the mechanisms by which factors such as age and biochemical status affect chemosensory preference. Because there is evidence to show age-related increases in olfactory and taste thresholds [see ref. 42–44 for a review], one could make the case that older people's preferences for higher concentrations of amino acids reflect their diminished taste or olfactory sensitivity. The present study suggests that the elderly participants' higher preferred concentration of casein hydrolysate is not simply due to generally lower perceived intensity. However, lower concentrations of casein hydrolysate or of flavor components within the lower concentrations of casein hydrolysate may fall below a person's odor or taste threshold. Removing one or more flavor 'notes' from a complex olfactory-taste mixture by failing to exceed the individual's threshold for that note could dramatically alter its acceptability, independent of perceived intensity.

Conclusions

The present studies suggest the importance of considering the complex chemosensory mixture when studying the effects of aging on taste perception. These studies further suggest that aging alters not only chemosensory sensitivity, but also chemosensory preference. Finally, this research indicates that the interrelationship between chemosensory perception and nutrition in the geriatric population is an area which warrants further study.

References

1 Balogh, K.; Lelkes, K.: The tongue in old age. Geront. clin. *3:* suppl., pp. 38–54 (1961).
2 Bartoshuk, L. M.: Effects of aging on chemical senses. Proc. 5th Annu. Meet. Ass. for Chemoreception Sciences, Sarasota 1983.
3 Beauchene, R. E.; Davis, T. A.: The nutritional status of the aged in the USA. Age *2:* 23 (1979).
4 Bouliere, F.; Cendron, H.; Rapaport, A.: Modification avec l'age des seuils gustatifs de perception et de reconnaissance aux saveurs salée et sucre, chez l'homme. Gerontologia *2:* 104–112 (1958).
5 Bowman, B. B.; Rosenberg, I. H.: Assessment of the nutritional status of the elderly. Am. J. clin. Nutr. *35:* 1142–1151 (1982).
6 Brownell, K. D.: Obesity: understanding and treating a serious, prevalent, and refractory disorder. J. consult. clin. Psychol. *50:* 820–840 (1982).
7 Cain, W. S.; Johnson, F.: Lability of odor pleasantness: influence of mere exposure. Perception *1:* 459–465 (1978).
8 Chalke, H. D.; Dewhurst, J. R.: Accidental coal-gas poisoning. Br. med. J. *ii:* 915–917 (1957).
9 Cooper, R. M.; Bilash, I.; Zubeck, J. P.: The effect of age on taste sensitivity. J. Geront. *14:* 56–58 (1959).

10 Cowart, B. J.: Direct scaling of the intensity of basic tastes: a life span study. 5th Annu. Meet. Ass. for Chemoreception Sciences, Sarasota 1983.

11 Desor, J. A.; Green, L. S.; Maller, O.: Preferences for sweet and salty tastes in 9- to 15-year-old and adult humans. Science 190: 686–687 (1975).

12 Dye, C. J.; Koziatek, D. A.: Age and diabetes effects on threshold and hedonic perception of sucrose solutions. J. Geront. 36: 310–315 (1981).

13 Engen, T.: The potential usefulness of odor and taste in keeping children away from harmful substances. Ann. N. Y. Acad. Sci. 237: 224–228 (1974).

14 Engen, T.: The perception of odors (Academic Press, New York 1982).

15 Enns, M. P.; Van Itallie, T. B.; Grinker, J. A.: Contributions of age, sex and degree of fatness on preferences and magnitude estimation for sucrose in humans. Physiol. Behav. 22: 999–1003 (1979).

16 Fordyce, I. D.: Olfaction tests. Br. J. Ind. Med. 18: 213–215 (1961).

17 Glanville, E. V.; Kaplan, A. R.; Fischer, R.: Age, sex and taste sensitivity. J. Geront. 19: 474–478 (1964).

18 Grzegorczyk, P. B.; Jones, S. W.; Mistretta, C. M.: Age-related differences in salt taste acuity. J. Geront. 34: 834–840 (1979).

19 Harris, H.; Kalmus, H.: The measurement of taste sensitivity to phenylthiourea (PTC). Ann. hum. Genet. 15: 24–31 (1949).

20 Hinchcliffe, R.: Clinical quantitative gustometry. Acta oto-lar. 49: 453–466 (1958).

21 Hinchcliffe, R.: Aging and sensory thresholds. J. Geront. 17: 45–50 (1962).

22 Hughes, G.: Changes in taste sensitivity with advancing age. Gerontologia Clinica 2: 224–230 (1969).

23 Hyde, R. J.; Feller, R. P.: Age and sex effects on taste of sucrose, NaCl, citric acid and caffeine. Neurobiol. Aging 2: 315–318 (1981).

24 Jansen, C.; Harrill, I.: Intakes and serum levels of protein and iron for 70 elderly women. Am. J. clin. Nutr. 30: 1414–1422 (1977).

25 Joyner, R. E.: Olfactory acuity in an industrial population. J. occup. Med. 5: 37–42 (1963).

26 Kalmus, H.; Trotter, W. R.: Direct assessment of the effect of age on PTC sensitivity. Ann. hum. Genet. 26: 145–149 (1962).

27 Kaplan, A.; Glanville, E.; Fischer, R.: Cumulative effect of age and smoking on taste sensitivity in males and females. J. Geront. 20: 334–337 (1965).

28 Kimbrell, G. M.; Furchtgott, E.: The effect of aging on olfactory threshold. J. Geront. 18: 364–365 (1963).

29 Laird, D. A.; Breen, W. J.: Sex and age alterations in taste preferences. J. Am. diet. Ass. 15: 549–550 (1939).

30 Langen, M. J.; Yearick, E. S.: The effects of improved oral hygiene on taste perception and nutrition of the elderly. J. Geront. 31: 413–418 (1976).

31 Lindgarde, F.; Malmquist, J.; Balke, B.: Physical fitness, insulin secretion, and glucose tolerance in healthy males and mild type 2 diabetes. Acta diabet. lat. 20: 33–40 (1983).

32 Martin, J. E.; Dubbert, P. M.: Exercise applications and promotion in behavioral medicine: current status and future direction. J. consult. clin. Psychol. 50: 1004–1007 (1982).

33 Minz, A. I.: Condition of the nervous system in old men. Z. Alternsforsch. 21: 271–277 (1968).

34 Moncrieff, R. W.: Odour preferences (Wiley, New York 1966).

35 Moore, L. M.; Nielson, C. R.; Mistretta, C. M.: Sucrose taste thresholds: age-related differences. J. Geront. 37: 64–69 (1982).

36 Moskowitz, H. R.; Kumraiah, V.; Sharma, K. N.; Jacobs, H. L.; Sharma, S. D.: Effects of hunger, satiety and glucose load upon taste intensity and taste hedonics. Physiol. Behav. *16:* 471–475 (1976).

37 Murphy, C.: The effects of age on taste sensitivity; *in* Han, Coons, Special senses in aging, pp. 21–33 (University of Michigan Institute of Gerontology, Ann Arbor 1979).

38 Murphy, C.: Effects of aging on chemosensory perception of blended foods, 3rd Annu. Meet. of the Ass. for Chemoreception Sciences, Sarasota 1981.

39 Murphy, C.: Effects of exposure and context on hedonics of olfactory-taste mixtures; in Kuznicki, Johnson, Rutkiewic, Selected sensory methods: problems and approaches to measuring hedonics, ASTM STP 773, pp. 60–70 (Am. Soc. for Testing and Materials, Philadelphia 1982).

40 Murphy, C.: Age-related effects on the threshold, psychophysical function, and pleasantness of menthol. J. Geront. *38:* 217–222 (1983).

41 Murphy, C.: Cognitive and chemosensory influences on age-related changes in the ability to identify blended foods. J. Geront. *40:* 47–52 (1985).

42 Murphy, C.: Taste and smell in the elderly; in Meiselman, Rivlin, Clinical measurement of taste and smell (Macmillan, New York, in press).

43 Murphy, C.; Withee, J.: Age-related differences in the pleasantness of chemosensory stimuli. Psychol. Aging *1:* 312–319 (1986).

44 Murphy, C.; Withee, J.: Age and biochemical status predict preference for casein hydrolysate. J. Geront. *42:* 73–77 (1987).

45 Murphy, C.; Nunez, K.; Withee, J.; Jalowayski, A. A.: The effects of age, nasal airway resistance and nasal cytology on olfactory threshold for butanol. Chem. Senses *10:* 418 (1985).

46 Richter, C.; Campbell, K.: Sucrose taste thresholds of rats and humans. Am. J. Physiol. *128:* 291–297 (1940).

47 Schiffman, S. S.: Changes in taste and smell with age: psychophysical aspects; in Ordy, Brizzee, Sensory systems and communication in the elderly (Raven Press, New York 1979).

48 Schiffman, S. S.; Clark, T. B.: Magnitude estimates of amino acids for young and elderly subjects. Neurobiol. Aging *1:* 81–91 (1980).

49 Schiffman, S. S.; Hornak, K.; Reilly, D.: Increased taste thresholds of amino acids with age. Am. J. clin. Nutr. *32:* 1622–1627 (1979).

50 Schiffman, S. S.; Moss, J.; Erickson, R. P.: Thresholds of food odors in the elderly. Exp. Aging Res. *2:* 389–398 (1976).

51 Schiffman, S. S.; Lindley, M. G.; Clark, T. B.; Makins, C.: Molecular mechanism of sweet taste: relationship of hydrogen bonding to taste sensitivity in both young and elderly. Neurobiol. Aging *2:* 173–185 (1981).

52 Smith, S. E.; Davies, P. D.: Quinine taste thresholds: a family study and a twin study. Ann. hum. Genet. *37:* 227–232 (1973).

53 Stevens, J. C.; Marks, L. E.: Cross-modality matching functions generated by magnitude estimation. Percept. Psychophys. *27:* 379–389 (1980).

54 Stevens, J. C.; Bartoshuk, L. M.; Cain, W. S.: Chemical senses and aging: taste versus smell. Chem. Senses *9:* 167–179 (1984).

55 Stevens, J. C.; Plantinga, A.; Cain, W. S.: Reduction of odor and nasal pungency associated with aging. Neurobiol. Aging *3:* 125–132 (1982).

56 Strauss, E. L.: A study on olfactory acuity. Ann. Otol. Rhinol. Lar. *79:* 95–104 (1970).

57 Venstrom, D.; Amoore, J. E.: Olfactory threshold in relation to age, sex or smoking. J. Food Sci. *33:* 264–265 (1968).

58 Weiffenbach, J. M.; Baum, B. J.; Burghauser, R.: Taste thresholds: quality specific
    variation with human aging. J. Geront. *37:* 700–706 (1982).
59 Wilkins, L.; Richter, C. P.: A great craving for salt by a child with cortico-adrenal
    insufficiency. J. Am. med. Ass. *114:* 866–868 (1940).
60 Yearick, E. S.; Wang, M. L.; Pisias, S. J.: Nutritional status of the elderly: dietary and
    biochemical findings. J. Geront. *35:* 663–671 (1980).

Dr. Claire Murphy, Department of Psychology, San Diego State University,
San Diego, CA 92182-0350 (USA)

Front. oral Physiol., vol. 6, pp. 151–167 (Karger, Basel 1987)

Taste Perception Mechanisms

James M. Weiffenbach

Clinical Investigations and Patient Care Branch, National Institute of Dental
Research, National Institutes of Health, Bethesda, Md., USA

Introduction

Taste is a major oral sensory system. Thus, defining the effects of age
on taste plays a key role in understanding the aging mouth. The measurement of age effects on taste perception, however, is complicated by the
very real possibility that performance differences in taste testing tasks
arise from non-sensory differences between age groups. This com-
plication challenges the psychophysicist and has stimulated refinements of
measurement technique that can be applied in other contexts. Moreover,
studies of taste in the elderly have documented alterations of function
that may be different in kind from those associated with systemic disease,
irradiation or drugs and thus may force a reexamination of our understanding of taste mechanisms [35]. Interestingly, the contribution that developmental studies of taste can make to gerontology, psychophysics and
the chemoreception sciences is quite independent of whether or not the
subjective appreciation of taste stimuli changes with age. It is potentially
as informative to document the circumstances under which subjective responses are maintained into advanced years as it is to chart the parallel
decline of subjective and objective indices of function.

The study of taste in aging encompasses more than the comparison of
an older and a younger group on an isolated measure of tasting. As in any
study of aging, the effects of increased age are to be isolated from effects
reflecting the increased incidence of disease and increased use of medications that sometimes accompany aging. Various parameters of age-
related change should be explored. The time course of performance
change is one such parameter. A function that begins to decline in middle
age should be discriminated from one that remains intact among all but
the extremely old. Age effects may also differ with respect to their generality in the population. A change in average values may reflect a weak
influence effecting a broad spectrum of the elderly or a marked effect

limited to some subgroup of the population. Additionally, aging may affect the taste system as a whole or portions of it specialized for particular taste qualities.

Defining Taste Mechanisms

The study of taste in aging is complicated by the fact that tasting involves the cooperative functioning of several distinct sensory systems each of which might undergo independent change across the life span. Taste, as it is commonly experienced, incorporates input from the oral taste receptors along with input from other oral and extra-oral sensory systems. Among the oral sensory systems are those for temperature, touch, pain (oral trigeminal) and the sensory-motor mechanisms involved in manipulating substances in the mouth. These systems combine with others to produce the subjective impressions of bulk, slickness, dryness, wetness and crispness that are elicited along with taste during eating. The interaction of these oral sensory systems with taste is little understood. A beginning, however, has been made. For example, oral trigeminal stimulation reduces sensitivity to some taste qualities [16] and stimulus variations that increase viscosity decrease the perceived sweetness of sugar and perceived saltiness of sodium chloride [7]. The mechanisms and age relations of these phenomena remain to be demonstrated. Taste experience is also modulated by the activity of extra-oral sensory systems. Perhaps the most notable effects are from nasal sensory systems. Airborne olfactory and trigeminal stimuli reach sensors in the nose either directly, via the nares, or indirectly, through the nasopharynx. Effects of aging on responses to nasal stimulation are well documented [see Murphy, this volume]. The demonstration that younger individuals lose their performance advantage over older individuals on a food recognition task if both groups occlude their nasal airway suggests that declining sensitivity to nasal stimuli might account for some reports of age associated taste changes [27].

In general, the definition of age-related changes is vastly complicated by the vulnerability of taste perception to changes in various nontaste sensory systems. When the focus of aging studies is upon taste mechanisms per se, the effects of possible age-related changes in the other sensory systems involved in taste perception can be mitigated by judicious selection of test stimuli. To obtain information directly relevant to oral taste system alterations, the stimuli should be well defined, simple, of neutral texture and presented at a uniform temperature. As far as possible, they should lack olfactory and trigeminal components and present no special problems of oral manipulation for either young or old individuals. This usually means aqueous solutions of substances representing the four basic taste qualities.

The definition of aging effects on taste is complicated not only by the interaction of the taste system with other sensory systems but by possible age-related alterations of the salivary milieu in which tasting occurs. The sensitivity of lingual taste receptors depends upon their adaptation to background stimuli. Indeed, studies of adaptation provide the essential evidence that the phenomonological division of taste experience into salty, sour, sweet, and bitter reflects four separate sensory mechanisms. Specifically, preexposure to stimuli representing one of the four basic taste qualities reduces sensitivity to other stimuli which elicit that quality without reducing sensitivity to stimuli eliciting other taste qualities [17, 19, 32]. Adaptation mechanisms directly relevant to salivary effects on taste have been demonstrated. Preexposure to an aqueous salt solution at the salinity of saliva decreases sensitivity to subsequent test samples of salt solutions; rinsing away the background of saliva increases measured sensitivity relative to assessments without a prestimulus rinse of distilled water [18]. Since saliva can act as an adapting stimulus, age-related changes affecting either saliva or the adaptation of taste receptors to it could alter taste experience. Although present evidence suggests that salivary output does not change markedly with age [Baum, this volume], taste adaptation may be sensitive to changes in salivary composition, buffering capacity or the temporal pattern of secretion which have not been studied in relation to age. Possible effects of age on the process of adaptation to taste stimuli are unexplored. Studies directed toward isolating the effects of age on tasting can, however, minimize salivary effects by using an oral rinse with distilled water before each sampling of test stimuli.

Mechanisms of Age-Related Change

Effects of age upon taste perception might arise from age effects on the anatomy of the taste system. In humans the taste end organs, or taste buds, are found in fungiform papillae on the lateral portions of the anterior dorsal tongue, in the circumvallate papillae on the posterior dorsal surface and in the slit like foliate papillae located on the posterior lateral aspect of the tongue. Fungiform papillae contain from zero to fifteen taste buds. Among taste bud-bearing fungiform papillae, the average number of buds is just over four [3]. Circumvallate papillae have an average number of taste buds in the range of 100–200. Foliate papillary ridges may likewise contain more than one hundred buds [24]. Other taste buds are located throughout the oral cavity, most notably at the junction of the hard and soft palate. It is believed that there are chemosensitive receptors on the epiglottis. Age effects on the peripheral anatomy of the taste system might include changes in the number or morphology of taste buds. Marked decreases in the number of taste buds with age have been found in mice [9a]. Recent studies have, however, failed to substantiate declines in taste bud number with age in rodents. Mistretta and Baum [21] found no significant difference in taste bud number for circumvallate papillae between young (6-month) and old (24-month) Wistar-derived rats. Mistretta and Oakley [22] found no significant difference between young (4- to 6-month) and older (20- to 24-month) Fischer 344 rats with respect to the percentage of fungiform papillae that contained the characteristic single taste bud. In animals 30–37 months of age, the percentage of taste bud-bearing papillae showed a slight but significant decline from 99.3 to 94.7%. The actual numbers of buds lost with age was very small. Bradley et al. [5a], studying the tongues of 15 adult rhesus monkeys between 4 and 31 years of age, found no age-related differences in the number of taste buds for any of the three gustatory papillae types and no alteration in taste bud diameter. Early studies of human cadavers supported an hypothesis of decreased taste bud number in old age for circumvallate papillae [1, 23] and for foliate papillae [23]. In the best designed and most recent study of human tongues, however, counts of taste buds in fungiform papillae failed to confirm the suggestion that advancing age is associated with decreased taste bud number [2].

Ideally, the investigation of aging in the taste system would involve a demonstration of correlated changes in anatomy and function. The study of age-related change in function need not, however, await the demonstration of effects of aging on taste system anatomy. Even if changes in peripheral anatomy were the underlying cause of altered taste function, currently available morphological techniques may not be sufficiently discriminating to demonstrate them. Current morphological techniques cannot, for example, discriminate between end organs responsible for different taste qualities. Although various areas in the mouth are differentially sensitive to the four taste qualities [9, 14], correlated differences in taste buds have not been demonstrated. Even the demonstration that individual papillae are differentially sensitive to the four taste qualities [6, 29] has not led to an identification of end organs responsive to particular qualities. It may be significant that these studies were carried out on young adults. Variation in sensitivity across areas or between papillae in young individuals may, in fact, not be reflected morphologically. Age-related dysfunction may be of a different nature. Variations in sensitivity due to aging may be correlated with morphological change. Indeed, an age-associated change in sensitivity that was specific to a particular quality might lead to the identification of an anatomical substrate for that quality. Thus, at present, studies of taste function in aging may have more to offer to the study of taste anatomy than vice versa.

The hypothesis that age-related changes in taste function arise from alterations in the peripheral end organs is not necessarily limited to morphological considerations. An end organ hypothesis might encompass alterations other than changes in the number and form of taste buds. One might imagine, for example, that changes in taste perception are related to altered turnover rates of taste cells, to changes in the number or affinity of critical cell surface receptors, or to changes in the permeability of taste cell membranes. In fact, it is not unreasonable to suggest that demonstrations establishing the relation of these cellular mechanisms to taste reception might be initially worked out within the context of aging research.

Assessing Taste Function

The assessment of taste function might be most directly approached by asking individuals to describe their taste experience. Each person does, after all, know their own sensory experience in a way that no one else can. Moreover, subjective reports may contain critical information that current objective measurement techniques ignore. The validity of subjective reports may be questioned. Problems of validity are magnified when comparisons across the life span are attempted. Strategies for developmental comparisons of subjective reports comprise several unattractive alternatives. Individuals differing in age might be asked to describe their own current inner experience of taste and the reports compared. Such comparisons are, however, suspect because descriptions generated by younger and older individuals might differ as a result of influences unrelated to taste function. Alternatively, older individuals might be asked to compare their current experience with their memory of past experiences. Retrospective comparisons are risky at best. They are particularly dangerous when they rely on the recollections of individuals whose memory functions may be impaired. Moreover, the actual stimuli eliciting the taste experiences may be different. The nursing home resident's subjective impression of taste loss may have nothing to do with psychological factors such as memory distortion. It might simply reflect real stimulus differences between the institutional food being consumed today and the home cooking of ten years ago. Bringing healthy, community-dwelling individuals of different ages into the same laboratory setting and having them respond to the same well characterized stimuli overcomes this particular problem.

Laboratory testing with modern psychophysical methods does more than just insure that the stimuli presented to older and younger individuals are standardized. In such a setting objective tests can be applied. Objective assessment techniques require that subjects prove that some specific aspect of stimulus information is available to them. In contrast, subjective techniques, whether in the laboratory or other settings, assume that subjects can and will give a valid report of their sensory experience. The difference between subjective and objective assessment can be highlighted by comparing alternative procedures for measuring the taste threshold, that stimulus strength which separates stronger stimuli that can be sensed from weaker ones that cannot. The critical element differentiating subjective assessment from objective assessment is the way the investigator views the subject's responses. Subjective techniques such as the yes/no procedure take the subject's response at face value. In a yes/no procedure subjects indicate whether or not individual test stimuli elicit a taste. When the subject responds 'no', the investigator infers that the stimulus did not elicit a taste. The subject's response, however, depends not only on the experience elicited by the stimulus but also on the subject's criterion for deciding what is and what is not enough of a sensation to report. This is a particularly severe problem for aging studies because age cohorts may differ systematically in their willingness to acknowledge a given level of experience as a taste. In contrast, objective techniques require subjects to demonstrate that they have received stimulus information by performing a task based on information available in the test stimulus. As an example, forced-choice threshold techniques present the subject two or more stimuli, all but one of which are blanks (distilled water), and require the subject to indicate which one has a taste. Even if none of the stimuli elicit a sensation meeting the subject's criterion for being called a taste, the subject must choose one alternative anyway. When the stimulus is above threshold, the task is performed without error. When the stimulus is below threshold, subjects do only as well as they could by chance alone.

Threshold Sensitivity

Attending to such niceties of measurement as requiring a prestimulus rinse and employing an objective assessment procedure does make a difference in aging studies. Early studies of taste thresholds used yes/no procedures and usually failed to incorporate a rinse to minimize effects of salivary adaptation [5, 10, 15, 26, 28]. All these studies demonstrated decreases in threshold sensitivity with age, but differences between the studies were large relative to the observed age effects. Subsequent studies [4, 13, 25, 36] using forced-choice procedures and prestimulus rinsing also found significant decrements in sensitivity with aging. Threshold differences between studies were, however, smaller. As detailed below, analysis of variance (ANOVA) yielded no significant differences in average thresholds for the same substance obtained from comparable young subjects in different studies. Age effects from different studies are referred to comparable baseline sensitivity. Thus, the examination of gerontological and psychophysical issues which follows is simplified. Issues include the quality specificity of effects as well as their generality across samples and the robustness with variation in experimental design. Another issue of gerontological concern involves a complex of influences that appears to be associated with living in residential care facilities.

Grzegorczyk et al. [13], Moore et al. [25], Weiffenbach et al. [36] and Bartoshuk et al. [4] each employed a distilled water rinse and the same two-alternative forced-choice detection task. The stimulus substances for sweet, salty, and sour were the same, although different quinine compounds were used for bitter. Bartoshuk et al. [4] and Weiffenbach et al. [37] used the up-down transformed method [38] to determine the progression of test stimulus concentrations and to calculate thresholds. A slight variant of this procedure was used in the other two studies. All in all, these studies are remarkably homogeneous in taste assessment methodology, but represent real differences in design strategy. They offer an unparalled opportunity to examine the generality of age effects and will be explored in some detail.

Three of these studies report detection thresholds for sodium chloride. These studies differed in design but yielded remarkably congruent findings. Grzegorczyk et al. [13] obtained thresholds for salt but for no other substances from 76 nonhospitalized subjects between the age of 23 and 93. The sex distribution of this sample was unspecified. Weiffenbach et al. [36] obtained salt thresholds along with thresholds for sweet, sour and bitter substances during the same tasting session. Thresholds were reported for 42 men and 39 women between 23 and 88 years of age who were community-dwelling, generally healthy, volunteer participants in the National Institute on Aging's, Baltimore Longitudinal Study of Aging. This sample was subsequently augmented with additional subjects from the same source to yield a final sample of 76 men and 69 women. Bartoshuk et al. [4] used a two-group design. A younger group made up of 16 women and 2 men of age 20–30 years was contrasted with 16 women and 2 men between 74 and 93 years old who were residents of a home for the elderly. Bartoshuk et al. [4] obtained thresholds for the different qualities on separate days. An ANOVA of salt thresholds obtained in these three studies from subjects matched in age to the younger group of Bartoshuk et al. [4] (i.e. age less than 31) yielded no significant difference between studies. While each of these three studies began from an equivalant baseline and each found a significant influence of age, different studies measured the effect of age differently. Bartoshuk et al. [4] reported a significant difference by nonparametric test between her two groups. Grzegorczyk et al. [13] reported a significant regression of threshold on age. They also plotted the rise in the percentage of individuals in each 20-year age bracket with thresholds above the average threshold for individuals under forty and contrasted the average thresholds of those under 40 with those over 65. Weiffenbach et al. [36] reported an age by sex ANOVA with three levels of age (below 45, 46 to 65, 66 and above). This analysis yielded a significant main effect for age in the absence of either a sex effect or an age by sex interaction. They also reported regression analyses that likewise reflect the influence of age, the absence of an overall threshold difference between men and women and the parallel effect of age on the sexes, findings which have been confirmed by analyses of the augmented sample. The age effect for salt thresholds is clearly robust with respect to variation in analytic strategy, age distribution, as well as the sex and institutional status of the subjects.

Bartoshuk et al. [4] and Weiffenbach et al. [36] each reported thresholds for a bitter tasting quinine compound from individuals from whom they had obtained other thresholds. In each study the effect of age was significant for both the quinine compound and for sodium chloride. Moreover, each study reported thresholds for some substance that did not yield a significant age effect. Bartoshuk et al. [4] found no age effect for 6-*n*-propylthiouracil (PROP), a bitter tasting substance for which a separate bitter mechanism has been proposed. Weiffenbach et al. [36] found no age effect for sucrose or citric acid. The absence of an age effect for even a single substance demonstrates that older subjects can perform the measurement task adequately and implies that the observed deficits reflect a sensory rather than a cognitive or attentional loss. Therefore, the decreased threshold sensitivity to bitter tasting quinine compounds or to salt observed in these two studies cannot be attributed to any difficulties the elderly might have in performing the threshold measurement task or to an across the board decrease in sensitivity to taste.

Weiffenbach et al. [36] obtained thresholds for all four qualities during a single session whereas Bartoshuk et al. [4] obtained thresholds for different qualities on different days. Moore et al. [25] obtained only one threshold from each subject. Their procedures, however, matched those used by Grzegorcyzk et al. [13] to assess salt sensitivity in subject from a roughly similar population. An ANOVA comparing the sucrose thresholds of individuals less than 31 years old from these three studies demonstrated no significant effects. Although, the baseline thresholds for young individuals did not differ, the reported effects of age did. Moore et al. [25] reported a significant regression of sucrose thresholds on age for the total sample and a significant group difference between thresholds for subgroups of subjects 20–45 and 60–80 years old. Bartoshuk et al. [4] reported a significant difference between average thresholds for their two age groups. In contrast, Weiffenbach et al. [36] found no significant increase in sucrose threshold with age. Neither ANOVA nor regression analyses yielded evidence of a significant influence of age or differential influence of age for the sexes. Analyses of the augmented sample yielded similar results. The clear difference between the sucrose findings of the several studies contrasts sharply with the uniformity of the findings for salt and for the quinine stimuli.

Weiffenbach et al. [36] found that sucrose thresholds showed no age effect, while thresholds obtained from the same individuals for other qualities did. This finding argues for a separate effect of aging on the taste mechanisms underlying different qualities. It is important to note that differential effects of other types can also support such a position. The sugar and salt thresholds reported by Bartoshuk et al. [4] provide an example. An ANOVA of these data yielded two significant effects: (1) a main effect for age that reflects the previously reported finding, and (2) a significant interaction of age with quality that is not apparent in the published report. Sucrose sensitivity declined less markedly with age than sensitivity to salt. This differential effect is in the same direction as the one reported by Weiffenbach et al. [36] and, like it, suggests that sucrose sensitivity is less vulnerable to the effects of age than is salt sensitivity. This type of interaction was not, however, found in an ANOVA using sucrose thresholds from Moore et al. [25] and salt thresholds from Grzegorczyk et al. [13]. As previously suggested [34], the failure to find a differential effect of age may be due to limited practice provided by the short session length of these two studies. Limitation on practice may affect older subjects more dramatically than younger ones. A comparison of sucrose and salt thresholds across the testing session presented by Moore et al. [25] shows a sharper rise in measured sensitivity for older (60–88 years of age) as compared to younger (20–45 years age) subjects. Moreover, differences between threshold for the age groups decreased more rapidly with experience for sucrose than for salt. This suggests that the sucrose threshold difference reported by Moore et al. [25] have a less substantial sensory base than the salt threshold differences obtained by Grzeorczyk et al. [13]. It may also be significant that these sucrose and salt thresholds were obtained from different subjects and that these subjects were drawn from different populations. The design of these studies exercises weaker control over both population differences and the differential effects of practice on older subjects than the other two studies providing a comparison of sucrose and salt sensitivity.

The citric acid thresholds obtained by Weiffenbach et al. [36], like the sucrose thresholds obtained from the same subjects, do not vary significantly with age. No influence of age was found for men or women alone, although the women were significantly more sensitive than the men. In contrast, Bartoshuk et al. [4] reported a significant difference between thresholds for older and younger subjects that remains significant if the 2 males in each sample are excluded. An ANOVA of the citric acid thresholds obtained from all the female subjects of these two studies and a similar one employing all 32 female subjects of Baroshuk et al. [4] but only the 16 oldest and youngest female subjects of Weiffenbach et al. [36] concurred in finding a highly significant interaction of age with study. The finding of an age effect for citric acid in the sample tested by Bartoshuk et al. [4] and not in that tested by Weiffenbach et al. [36] may represent a population difference, perhaps one based on residence in an institution or on oral health status changes associated with institutionalization.

Intensity Perception

Although most laboratory studies of taste and aging have used thresholds to assess taste function, the relevance of threshold sensitivity to tasting experience is open to question. Threshold change provides a severely limited mechanism for the reported taste complaints of the elderly [8]. Although substantial elevations of threshold might account for failures to detect the saltiness or bitterness of foods, most real life alterations in taste may not be absolute failures to detect weak tastes but rather decreases in the perceived intensity of stimuli that are detected. The perception of the intensity of stimuli above threshold can be quantified by modern psychophysical techniques of direct scaling.

Direct scaling procedures require subjects to make judgments of relative strength. If one stimulus is twice as strong as another, the response to it should be twice as large. A taste that is a third as strong as another should get a response one third as large. In early direct scaling studies, a standard stimulus with an investigator assigned value, called the modulus, was presented along with a test stimulus each time the subject made a judgment. For example, the subject might be presented with the modulus with a value of 10 and then a comparison stimulus. A subject who perceived the test stimulus as twice as strong as the modulus should assign it a 20. Experience showed that subjects did just as well if, the modulus, rather than being presented on each trial, was presented periodically throughout a session or only once at the beginning. In fact, it is not necessary to have a modulus at all. In the modulus free variant of direct scaling, subjects are apparently able to use their response to the first stimulus as a self-assigned modulus or to judge each stimulus in relation to the preceding one.

Three variants of direct scaling have been used in the study of taste intensity perception in aging. All require ratio judgments but each uses a different approach to providing comparability between responses generated by older and younger subjects (e.g. controlling for differences in the way older and younger subjects approach the task). In the direct scaling procedure termed magnitude estimation, subjects generate numbers to represent ratios between perceived intensities. Magnitude estimation is suspect to the degree that different age cohorts use numbers differently. Some differences between individuals or groups are analogous to modulus differences and these can be compensated for by mathematical transformation of the subject's responses. If one subject responds to a moderate stimulus with a 5 and to a stronger one with a 10 whereas another subject responds to these stimuli with a 50 and a 100, the parallel nature of their responding can be highlighted by normalization which brings the average magnitude scores to a common value by multiplying the responses of each subject by an appropriate factor. In the example given above, all the first subject's responses could be multiplied by 10 and all the other subject's by one. This compensates for differences in the size of the numbers but leaves the ratio properties of the subjects' judgments intact. Another variant of direct scaling, magnitude matching, makes special provision for defining a normalization factor. In magnitude matching, magnitude estimates (numbers) are obtained for stimuli of two sensory modalities during the same session. For example, intensity judgments of auditory stimuli have been used to obtain a normalization factor for taste intensity judgments. Multiplication by this factor brings the scores of an individual whose concept of numbers causes him to give numerically large estimates of intensity for both tones and tastes into register with an individual who uses small numbers for both. Either of these individuals can be discriminated from a subject with a taste loss who uses systematically smaller numbers for taste than for tone.

Cross-modality matching provides a more direct escape from dependence on number concepts. Cross-modal matching allows subjects to indicate their responses by adjusting the magnitude of a variable sensory stimulus, as by adjusting the brightness of a light, the loudness of a sound or by generating a distance in space. Concepts of loudness or spatial extent are perhaps less likely than number concepts to differ systematically with age.

The usual analysis of direct scaling data specifies the relation of ratio intensity judgments to some physical measure of stimulus strength. Numbers reflecting intensity judgments and stimulus strength are both converted to logarithms and judged intensity plotted against physical strength to yield a psychophysical function. Then a least squares regression technique is used to calculate the slope of the best fitting straight line. The slope of the regression line provides a reasonably good characterization of the psychophysical function for those sensory modalities, including taste, that conform to the power law of Stevens [33]. The potential for comparing younger and older individuals with respect to the slope of the psychophysical function representing the rise in perceived intensity with taste stimulus concentration has in fact been exploited only recently.

Schiffman and Clark [30] had 41 male and 69 female college students and 42 female nursing home residents of unspecified age scale a variety of complex taste stimuli. Schiffman et al. [31] obtained magnitude estimates for 10 artificial sweeteners from 9 women and 3 men between 18 and 26 years of age and from 10 women and 1 man who ranged in age from 74 to 82. In each study, visual inspection showed that slopes of the group functions for older subjects were flattened relative to those obtained from the college age group. The ratio between the slopes for the younger and older groups exceeded unity for each taste substance. Enns et al. [11] obtained magnitude estimates for aqueous solutions of sucrose from children (n = 21), college students (n = 27) and elderly subjects (n = 17). They analyzed the logarithm of intensity judgments by ANOVA and found a significant interaction of age with stimulus concentration. They concluded that the rise in response magnitude with concentration for the college student and the elderly groups did not differ and that the sharper increase of ratings with concentration for the children accounted for the significant ANOVA finding. The clear implication is that the psychophysical function for the two older groups was flattened relative to that of the children.

Three studies of aging have obtained direct scaling responses for stimuli representing each of the four basic tastes. Bartoshuk et al. [4] compared the intensity judgments of 16 women and 2 men between the ages of 20 and 30 with similar responses obtained from 16 women and 2 men of 74–93 years of age. Taste intensity judgments, expressed in numbers, were normalized to each subject's intensity judgments of noise. For each quality, the slope of the older group was flattened relative to that of the younger group. Cowart [10a], sampling the age range systemically, obtained ratio scaling of intensity by cross-modal matching from 12 subjects in each of the following six age groups: 4–6, 10–12, 19–22, 35–44, 55–67, and 75–98 years of age. Each age group contained an equal number of males and females. Taste intensity judgments were expressed in terms of distances in space which the subject generated by extending the blade of a tape measure. Thus their judgments can be thought of as being normalized to judgments of spatial extent. For all qualities, the group slopes for older subjects were less steep than those generated by younger subjects. Weiffenbach et al. [37] also obtained crossmodal ratio judgments. Their subjects were 91 men and 79 women between the ages of 23 and 88. Groups of subjects 22–39, 40–56, 57–70 and over 70 contained approximately equal numbers of men and women. As in Cowart's study, subjects expressed their judgments in terms of spatial extent. Group functions for elderly individuals were flatter than those for younger persons. In each of the studies for which four quality comparisons are provided, log-log plots of response magnitude against stimulus concentration are presented for each quality. Considering only the results for roughly comparable age groups from Bartoshuk et al. [4] (20–30 and 74–93 years) from Cowart [10a] (19.6–22.6 and 71.5–93.3 years) and from Weiffenbach et al. [37] (22–39 and 71–88 years) leads to the conclusion that the rise in intensity with concentration is steeper for young adults than for the elderly. Going beyond this very limited conclusion is difficult. Considering the intermediate age groups of Cowart and Weiffenbach et al. suggests differences between the studies. Weiffenbach et al. [37] found that the group functions for any given quality were remarkably similar whether generated by the 40- to 56-year-olds, the 57- to 70-year-olds or those over 70. This suggests that age effects on those aspects of taste performance reflected in slope are essentially complete by age 40 and characterized by relative stability thereafter. Cowart, in contrast, found a systematic decline as a function of age for quinine sulfate slopes.

Detailed analyses of group psychophysical functions are ultimately unsatisfactory because there is no clearly appropriate test for the significance of difference in slope between group functions. As an alternative to an analysis based on group functions Weiffenbach et al. [37] calculated individual regression equations. Regression coefficients characterizing each subjects performance for each quality were analyzed by an age $\times$ sex $\times$ quality ANOVA. A significant effect for quality reflected the steeper slopes for sucrose and salt relative to citric acid and quinine sulfate. Importantly, neither the age main effects nor any interactions involving age were significant. Individual slopes, although appropriate to statistical test, demonstrated no significant age effects in this study.

Instead of characterizing intensity perception in terms of the slope of the best fitting regression line, one might examine other aspects of the psychophysical function. Changes in performance that flatten the slope of the function may, in fact, be better viewed as changes in the shape of the psychophysical function. Cowart [10a] found that for high stimulus concentrations the group curves for older subjects lay below those for younger subjects. Using a conservative test, she found statistically significant differences between the median responses of younger and older age groups at higher stimulus concentrations but no such differences at low concentrations. This finding was consistent for all four qualities and was also reflected in the data reported by Weiffenbach et al. [37]. In contrast, Bartoshuk et al. [4] found that the curves for the older group lay above that for the younger group at the lower concentrations and found significant differences between age group curves for lower but not for higher concentrations. This difference between the findings might reflect the free-living versus institutionalized status of the elderly subjects. Bartoshuk et al. [4], in fact, hypothesize a specific mechanism of shape distortion based on a mild dysgeusia or a chronic background taste in the mouth, associated with dental problems and poor oral hygiene of her population (see also Langan and Yearick, [15a]). This family of mechanisms are of gerontological interest. The shape of the functions generated by the elderly in each study are, however, quite similar. The curves for older subjects may simply be differentially displaced relative to those for younger subjects. Normalization provides vertical displacement that can make the same curve appear elevated at low concentrations, flattened at high concentrations or distorted at both low and high concentrations. To the degree that difference between the studies depends on differences in normalization, the resolution of these conflicting results is of importance to psychophysics.

Two measures of performance on the taste intensity judgment task which are alternative to the above analyses and are applicable to the assessment of individual performance have been explored by Cowart [10a] and Weiffenbach et al. [37] The reliability of a subject's discriminative responding over repeated trial was assessed using the intraclass correlation coefficient (ICC) while the monotonicity of individual psychophysical functions was assessed using Ferguson's [12] nonparametric test of trend. For each measure, a single score characterizes the performance of a subject in response to each quality. ICCs are derived from an ANOVA of raw sources and reflect the proportion of variation in an individual's judgments accounted for by variation in stimulus concentration. High

ICCs scores are obtained when there is close agreement between repeated judgments of the same concentration relative to the spread of judgments for different concentrations. Low ICCs indicate relative unreliability of response. On average, older subjects obtain lower ICCs than younger ones. Cowart and Weiffenbach et al. each found that ANOVA of ICCs yielded significant age effects for three of the four qualities. Within each study, one quality showed no age-related impairment. Thus, older individuals in each study were able to achieve ICC scores equivalent to those of younger persons. When lower average ICCs were obtained from the older subjects they reflected an impairment that was general in the sense that many of the older subjects demonstrated some impairment and no subgroup of markedly impaired individuals accounted for the observed shift in average values. In contrast, a small number of subjects are responsible for all the instances in which intensity judgments deviated significantly from a monotonic rise. Cowart [10a] reports that only five of the 48 subjects who rated all four qualities generated any trends which were nonmonotonic. Four failed to generate significant trend when rating quinine and one when rating citric acid. No subjects generated nonmonotonic trends for more than one quality. Four of the 5 subjects were male and 4 were over 55 years of age. Weiffenbach et al. [37] reported similar findings. Only 10 of their 170 subjects failed to generated significantly monotonic trend for all four qualities. Six of these 10 individuals were 70 years of age or older and only one was under 40. All but one were men. No individual failed to generate monotonic trend for more than one quality. Failure to generate monotonic trend likely reflects a specific breakdown of information transmission in the taste system rather than an inability to perform the scaling task. Failure of intensity judgments to reflect the ordering of the stimuli by concentration is rare, age-related and markedly more frequent in males than females. Its occurrence in individuals is quality-specific.

Conclusion

The present review demonstrates the degree of detail required to describe the taste functioning of the aging mouth. Age-related changes in taste perception are not uniform for all taste qualities, for all taste performances nor for all populations of elderly individuals. Each of the objective measures of age-related taste performance change shows some degree of quality specificity. This specificity implies both that the mechanisms underlying the four basic taste qualities age independently and that observed deficits reflect age-related sensory loss rather than age-related declines in the skills needed to perform the measurement task. Studies of aging demonstrate the separate variation of different aspects of taste functioning. For example, the capacity to detect weak taste stimuli shows a different pattern of age-related decline than does the capacity to appreciate increments in the intensity of stronger taste stimuli. Moreover, different parameters of a single performance may reflect different perceptual functions and display differential impairment with age as when the slopes of individual psychophysical functions did not show age effects but the reliability of intensity judgments do. Existing studies demonstrate the sensitivity of currently available objective measurement techniques to age-associated variation in taste functioning and provide ample evidence of a productive interaction between taste psychophysics and the study of aging.

References

1 Avey, L. B.; Tremaine, M. J.; Monzingo, F. L.: The numerical and topographical relations of circumvallate papillae throughout the life span. Anat. Rec. *64:* 9–25 (1935).
2 Arvidson, K.: Location and variation in number of taste buds in human fungiform papillae. Scand. J. dent. Res. *87:* 435–442 (1979).
3 Arvidson, K.; Friberg, U.: Human taste: response and taste bud number in fungiform papillae. Science *209:* 807–808 (1980).
4 Bartoshuk, L. M.; Rifkin, B.; Marks, L. E.; Bars, P.: Taste and aging. J. Geront. *41:* 51–57 (1986).
5 Bourliere, P. F.; Cendron, H.; Rapaport, A.: Modification avec l'âge des seuils gustatifs de perception et de reconnaissance aux saveurs salée et sucrée chez l'homme. Gerontologia *2:* 104–112 (1958).
5a Bradley, R. M.; Stedman, H. M.; Mistretta, C. M.: A quantitative study of lingual taste buds and papillae in the aging rhesus monkey tongue; in Davis, Leathers, Behavior and pathology of aging in rhesus monkeys (Alan Liss, New York 1985).
6 Cardello, A. V.: Chemical stimulation of single human fungiform taste papillae. Sensitivity profiles and locus of stimulation. Sens. Proc. *2:* 173–190 (1978).
7 Christensen, C. M.: Effects of solution viscosity on perceived saltiness and sweetness. Percept. Psychophys. *28:* 347–353 (1980).
8 Cohen, T.; Gitman, L.: Oral complaints and taste perception in the aged. J. Geront. *14:* 294–298 (1959).
9 Collings, V.: Human taste response as a function of locus of stimulation on the tongue and soft palate. Percept. Psychophys. *16:* 169–175 (1974).
9a Conger, A. D.; Wells, M. A.: Radiation and aging effects on taste structure and function. Rad. Res. *37:* 31–49 (1969).
10 Cooper, R. M.; Bilash, I.; Zubek, J. P.: The effect of age on taste sensitivity. J. Geront. *14:* 50–58 (1959).
10a Cowart, B. J.: Age-related changes in taste perception: direct scaling of intensity and pleasantness of basic tastes. PhD dissertation, The George Washington University, Washington D.C. (Sept. 1982).

11   Enns, M. P.; Van Itallie, J. B.; Grinker, J. A.: Contribution of age, sex, and degree
      of fatness on preferences and magnitude estimations of sucrose in humans. Physiol.
      Behav. *22:* 999–1003 (1979).
12   Ferguson, G. A.: Nonparametric trend analysis (McGill University Press, Montreal
      1965).
13   Grzegorczyk, P. B.; Jones, S. W.; Mistretta, C. M.: Age-related differences in salt
      taste acuity. J. Geront. *34:* 834–840 (1979).
14   Henkin, R. I.; Christiansen, R. I.: Taste evaluation on the tongue, palate, and
      pharynx of normal man. J. appl. Physiol. *22:* 316–320 (1967).
15   Hinchcliffe, R.: Clinical quantitative gustometery. Acta oto-lar. *49:* 453–466 (1958).
15a   Langan, M. J.; Yearick, E. S.: The effects of improved oral hygiene on taste percep-
      tion and nutrition of the elderly. J. Geront. *31:* 413–418 (1976).
16   Lawless, H.; Stevens, D. A.: Effects of oral chemical irritation on taste. Physiol. Be-
      hav. *32:* 995–998 (1984).
17   McBurney, D. H.: Gustatory cross adaptation between sweet-tasting compounds. Per-
      cept. Psychophys. *11:* 225–227 (1972).
18   McBurney, D.H.; Pfaffmann, C.: Gustatory adaptation to saliva and sodium chloride.
      J. exp. Psychol. *65:* 523–529 (1963).
19   McBurney, D. H.; Smith, D. V.; Shick, T. R.: Gustatory cross adaptation: sourness
      and bitterness. Percept. Pshchophys. *11:* 227–232 (1972).
20   Mistretta, C. M.: Aging effects on anatomy and neurophysiology of taste and smell.
      Gerodontology *3:* 131–136 (1984).
21   Mistretta, C. M.; Baum, B. J.: Quantitative study of taste buds in fungiform and
      circumvallate papillae of young and aged rats. J. Anat. *138:* 323–332 (1984).
22   Mistretta, C. M.; Oakley, I. A.: Quantitative anatomical study of taste buds in fungi-
      form papillae of young and old Fischer rats. J. Geront. *41:* 315–318 (1986).
23   Mochizuki, Y.: An observation on the numerical and topographical relations of taste
      buds to circumvallate papillae of Japanese. Okajimas Folia anat. jap. *15:* 595–608
      (1937).
24   Mochizuki, Y.: Studies on the foliate papillae of Japanese. 2. The number of taste
      buds. Okajimas Folia anat. jap. *18:* 355–369 (1939).
25   Moore, L. M.; Nielsen C. R.; Mistretta, C. M.: Sucrose taste thresholds: age-related
      differences. J. Geront. *37:* 64–69 (1982).
26   Murphy, C.: The effect of age in taste sensitivity; in Han, Coons, Special senses in
      aging: a current biological assessment (University of Michigan, Ann Arbor 1979).
27   Murphy, C.: Cognitive and chemosensory influences on age-related changes in the
      ability to identify blended foods. J. Geront. *40:* 47–52 (1985).
28   Richter, C. P.; Campbell, K. N.: Sucrose taste thresholds in rats and humans. Am. J.
      Physiol. *128:* 291–297 (1940).
29   Sandick, B.; Cardello, A. V.: Taste profiles from single circumvallate papillae: com-
      parison with fungiform profiles. Chem. Senses *6:* 197–214 (1981).
30   Schiffman, S. S.; Clark, J. R.: Magnitude estimates of amino acids for young and elder-
      ly subjects. Neurobiol. Aging *1:* 81–91 (1980).
31   Schiffman, S. S.; Lindley, M. G.; Clark, J. B.; Makin, C.: Molecular mechanisms of
      sweet taste: relationship of hydrogen bonding to taste sensitivity in both young and
      elderly. Neurobiol. Aging *64:* 153–181 (1981).
32   Smith, D. V.; McBurney, D. H.: Gustatory cross-adaptation: Does a single mechanism
      code the salty taste? J. exp. Psychol. *80:* 10–105 (1969).
33   Stevens, S. S.: On psychophysical law. Psychol. Rev. *64:* 153–181 (1957).
34   Weiffenbach, J. M.: Taste and smell perception in aging. Gerondontology *3:* 137–146
      (1984).

35   Weiffenbach, J. M.: Contributions from the study of development; in Meiselman, Rivi-
     lin, Clinical measurement of taste and smell, pp. 279–281 (Macmillan, New York
     1986).
36   Weiffenbach, J. M.; Baum, B. J.; Burghauser, R.: Taste thresholds. Quality specific
     variation with human aging. J. Geront. *37:* 372–377 (1982).
37   Weiffenbach, J. M.; Cowart, B. J.; Baum, B. J.: Taste intensity perception in aging. J.
     Geront. *41:* 460–468 (1986).
38   Wetherill, G. B.; Levitt, H. H.: Sequential estimations of points on a psychometric
     function. Br. J. Math. Stat. Psychol. *18:* 1–10 (1965).

James M. Weiffenbach, PhD Clinical Investigations and Patient Care Branch,
National Institute of Dental Research, National Institutes of Health,
Bethesda, MD 20892 (USA)

Subject Index

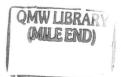